EXAMINATION SCHEMES IN GENERAL SURGERY AND ORTHOPAEDICS

i

EXAMINATION SCHEMES IN GENERAL SURGERY AND ORTHOPAEDICS

Chris Servant MB BS BSc (Hons) FRCS
Specialist Orthopaedic Registrar
The Royal United Hospital
Bath

Shaun Purkiss MS FRCS
Senior Lecturer
The Royal London Hospital
Whitechapel
London

G M M

© 1999

Greenwich Medical Media Ltd
219 The Linen Hall
162-168 Regent Street
London
W1R 5TB

ISBN: 1 900151 383

First Published 1999

Distributed worldwide by
Oxford University Press

Designed and Produced by
Diane Parker, Saldatore Limited

Printed in Great Britain by
Ashford Colour Press

CONTENTS

GLOSSARY OF ABBREVIATIONS vi
INTRODUCTION viii
EXAMINATION TECHNIQUE ix
SURGICAL HISTORY-TAKING xi
GENERAL PRINCIPLES OF CLINICAL EXAMINATION xii

SCHEMES IN GENERAL SURGERY

GENERAL SURGICAL SYMPTOMS 1
EXAMINATION OF A LUMP 3
EXAMINATION OF AN ULCER 5
EXAMINATION OF A NECK LUMP 7
EXAMINATION OF A THYROID LUMP 12
EXAMINATION OF THE BREAST 16
EXAMINATION OF THE CHEST 19
EXAMINATION OF THE ABDOMEN .23
EXAMINATION OF THE GROINS 28
RECTAL EXAMINATION 32
GENERAL EXAMINATION OF THE ARTERIOPATH 34
EXAMINATION OF VARICOSE VEINS .38

SCHEMES IN ORTHOPAEDICS

ORTHOPAEDIC SYMPTOMS 43
EXAMINATION OF A JOINT 45
EXAMINATION OF THE SHOULDER .48
EXAMINATION OF THE ELBOW 56
EXAMINATION OF THE WRIST 60
EXAMINATION OF THE HAND 65
EXAMINATION OF THE HIP 70
EXAMINATION OF THE KNEE 77
EXAMINATION OF THE ANKLE AND FOOT 85
EXAMINATION OF THE CERVICAL SPINE 92
EXAMINATION OF THE THORACOLUMBAR SPINE 99
EXAMINATION OF THE PERIPHERAL NERVOUS SYSTEM 106
EXAMINATION OF THE BRACHIAL PLEXUS 111
EXAMINATION OF PERIPHERAL NERVE LESIONS 115
EXAMINATION OF A MULTIPLE TRAUMA PATIENT 119
INDEX 127

GLOSSARY OF ABBREVIATIONS

ACJ . . . . .acromioclavicular joint
ACL . . . . .anteror cruciate ligament
AP . . . . .anteroposterior
ASIS . . . . .anterior superior iliac spine
BP . . . . .blood pressure
Ca . . . . .carcinoma
CMCJ . . . . .carpometacarpal joint
CT . . . . .computed tomography
CVA . . . . .cerebrovascular accident
CVP . . . . .central venous pressure
DIPJ . . . . .distal interphalangeal joint
DM . . . . .diabetes mellitus
ECG . . . . .electrocardiogram
ENT . . . . .ear, nose and throat
ETT . . . . .endotracheal tube
F_1O_2 . . . . .inspired fraction of oxygen
FBC . . . . .full blood count
FDP . . . . .flexor digitorum profundus
FDS . . . . .flexor digitorum superficialis (sublimis)
FH . . . . .family history
GT . . . . .greater trochanter
IPJ . . . . .interphalangeal joint
IV . . . . .intravenous
IVC . . . . .inferior vena cava
JVP . . . . .jugular venous pressure
LIF . . . . .left iliac fossa
LSV . . . . .long saphenous vein
LUQ . . . . .left upper quadrant
LVF . . . . .left ventricular failure
MCPJ . . . . .metacarpophalangeal joint
MTPJ . . . . .metatarsophalangeal joint
MI . . . . .myocardial infarction
MRCS .membership of the Royal College of Surgeons
MRI . . . . .magnetic resonance imaging
N . . . . .normal
O_2 . . . . .oxygen
OA . . . . .osteoarthritis
PA . . . . .posteroanterior
PIPJ . . . . .proximal interphalangeal joint
PMH . . . . .past medical history
PSIS . . . . .posterior superior iliac spine
R . . . . .rib
RA . . . . .rheumatoid arthritis
RIF . . . . .right iliac fossa
RUQ . . . . .right upper quadrant
SCJ . . . . .sternoclavicular joint
SFJ . . . . .saphenofemoral junction

SIJ . . . . .sacroiliac joint
SOB . . . . .shortness of breath
SSV . . . . .short saphenous vein
TB . . . . .tuberculosis
TIA . . . . .transient ischaemic attack
U&Es . . . . .urea and electrolytes
US . . . . .ultrasound scan
XR . . . . .X-ray film (radiograph)
1° . . . . .primary
2° . . . . .secondary
+ve . . . . .positive
–ve . . . . .negative
⇒ . . . . .implies, suggests

↑ . . . . .increased

↓ . . . . .decreased

Where an angle is recorded in brackets after a movement, it refers to the normal range
of the movement in a young adult.

INTRODUCTION

The Royal Colleges have introduced the MRCS Diploma to signify the successful completion of basic surgical training. This has replaced the FRCS Diploma, which is now awarded to those who have completed higher surgical training and are successful in the intercollegiate speciality examination.

The clinical section of the MRCS Examination, upon which this book focuses, consists of 'short cases' from all surgical specialities. It lasts a minimum of 40 minutes and the case mix encountered will be relevant to the whole syllabus.

The schemes presented in this book are an attempt to structure the examination of a region or specific entity into logical steps, such that the candidate can approach a patient's condition in a systematic manner. This will hopefully avoid a haphazard examination performance, which will always score poorly in British surgeons' eyes.

Each examination scheme is not intended to be a exhaustive description of the complete technique but should be used as an *aide-mémoire* to the candidate's own examination style. This should have been developed with experience over the course of the candidate's training. Constant repetition and personal observation of senior colleagues on the wards and in clinics, as well as from teaching received during postgraduate courses and from surgical tutors, is the secret of success.

Examination steps described in the sections headed 'Special tests' and 'Additional views' listed in the X-ray sections are further techniques that are not generally required at MRCS level but are included for completeness. They will be useful in daily clinical practice and will need to be known later at FRCS level.

Good luck!

Chris Servant and Shaun Purkiss
May 1998

EXAMINATION TECHNIQUE

The clinical section of the MRCS Examination consists of a broad range of surgical 'short cases'. At each examination centre there will be five separate areas or bays, with two examiners in each bay. In each bay a different part of the syllabus will be tested, as follows:

1. Identification of palpable or superficial lumps.
2. History and examination of the musculoskeletal system.
3. Assessment of the circulatory system.
4. Examination of the chest or abdomen.
5. Assessment of communication skills (e.g. explaining terminal disease, obtaining consent for a procedure).

In each of bays 1-4 three to five patients will be examined over 10 minutes. Fifteen minutes will be spent in bay 5, where a clinical scenario will be presented to the candidate, with an actor playing the part of a patient or relative.

A close marking system will be used in each bay and a pass in at least three bays will be required to pass overall. Borderline candidates will be discussed.

To be successful, a candidate must demonstrate a competent approach to the clinical assessment of a surgical patient. The examiners should get the impression that you always examine your patients in the same thoughtful and methodical manner. To this end the schemes presented in this book are aimed at helping candidates to develop a systematic and sympathetic examination technique.

On approaching a patient, listen carefully to the examiner's instructions. They are usually helpful and are rarely misleading. Introduce yourself to the patient and ask them to uncover the area to be examined. For most limb problems and for many other conditions (e.g. neck and breast pathology) it should be remembered that the other side is usually 'normal' and available for comparison. For example, if asked to examine the right wrist, ask the patient to show both wrists. Often re-examination of the abnormal side, after examining the normal side, serves to emphasize any positive findings. If the abnormal side is painful, examination of the normal side first gains the patient's confidence, allowing them to relax; this is important, for example, when examining the abdomen or when assessing joint stability.

Your examination technique should be well rehearsed and slick. Look at the patient rather than the examiners. Ask a few relevant questions as you proceed through your routine. An approach that shows a caring and sympathetic attitude is a prerequisite for all aspects of a clinical examination. You should also develop an easy rapport with the patient so that you gain their trust. Instances in which a patient suffers embarrassment, indignation or pain will score poorly and may possibly fail the candidate. As a consequence ask if there is any pain in an area about to be examined before palpating the area. In addition, if asked to examine the abdomen, groin or legs, try to be discrete about exposure of the external genitalia, unless this is a necessary part of the examination. The occasional brief pleasantry with the patient may be appropriate to keep them comfortable throughout their ordeal. As well as introducing yourself prior to starting, at the end of the examination you should thank the patient.

There are certain examination procedures, such as rectal examination, which should not be performed in the MRCS Examination. However, if they are relevant to the patient's condition, it will be expected that this is mentioned in your presentation of the examination findings.

It is important that you can demonstrate that you can think as you go along. You should express a desire to examine other systems if they are related to a clinical sign found in a local area. You should also look for clues away from the patient to deduce what is required of you. For instance, a glass of water indicates that you ought to examine for a thyroid swelling and plastic gloves suggest bimanual examination of the submandibular glands.

Some examiners like you to present your findings at the end of your examination of a patient. Other examiners prefer to have a running commentary during the examination process. This can be more difficult to do as thoughts, which are best contained, may slip out inadvertently. It is probably best to practice both the presentation and commentary styles for all systems before entering the examination.

After performing the examination the positive findings should be emphasized and the *relevant* negative findings presented efficiently. While presenting it is a good idea to look at the examiner's nose. This prevents you from being distracted and also, by avoiding adrenaline-affected eye contact, it will not intimidate the examiner unduly. The occasional glance to the patient emphasizes that you are talking about a human being and can add expression to a performance. Try to express yourself succinctly and clearly rather than rely on hand gestures to describe your findings.

When revising your examination techniques it is sensible to bear in mind that patients who turn up to the clinical section of the MRCS Examination usually have chronic problems that are easily demonstrated. For example, a reducible inguinal hernia is much more likely to present than acute appendicitis.

SURGICAL HISTORY-TAKING

The following scheme forms the basis of taking a comprehensive surgical history. In its entirety it would not be required for the clinical section of the MRCS Examination, which comprises only 'short cases'. However, it is a useful template for everyday clinical use and it also provides the background for the more succinct approach required for surgical short cases.

Patient details
- Name.
- Age.
- Gender.
- Occupation.
- Handedness (upper limb or cervical spine problems).

Presenting complaint
- General description of complaint (site, nature, onset, duration).
- Specific features of complaint.
- Remaining questions about abnormal system.

Systems
- Cardiorespiratory system (see **GENERAL SURGICAL SYMPTOMS,** page 1).
- Gastrointestinal system (see **GENERAL SURGICAL SYMPTOMS,** page1).
- Genitourinary system (see **GENERAL SURGICAL SYMPTOMS,** page 1).
- Endocrine system (see **EXAMINATION OF A THYROID LUMP,** page 12).
- Peripheral nervous system (see **ORTHOPAEDIC SYMPTOMS,** page 43).
- Musculoskeletal system (see **ORTHOPAEDIC SYMPTOMS,** page 43).

Past medical history
- Operations.
- Accidents.
- Illnesses.
- History of DM, TB, MI, CVA, hypertension, rheumatic fever, jaundice, asthma, epilepsy.

Family history
- Major hereditary conditions among relatives (e.g. family cancer syndromes).

Social history
- Activities of daily living.
- Smoking habits.
- Alcohol consumption.

Drug history
- Current medication.
- Known allergies.

GENERAL PRINCIPLES OF CLINICAL EXAMINATION

- Introduce yourself to the patient.
- Ask the patient for permission to perform an examination.
- Adequately expose the appropriate part (but exercise discretion if the external genitalia are to be exposed).
- Expose the 'normal' side for comparison, if relevant.
- Ask the patient if the area to be examined is painful.
- Look at the patient's expression throughout examination (to help in localizing pain and tenderness but do not hurt the patient unduly).

General surgery
- Inspection (look).
- Palpation (feel).
- Percussion (tap).
- Auscultation (listen).
- Imaging (X-ray).

Orthopaedics
- Inspection (look).
- Palpation (feel).
- Movement (move).
- Imaging (X-ray).

Additional tests/special tests
- Ask a few relevant questions during your examination.
- If relevant, mention to the examiners that you would normally perform a rectal examination and analyse the urine.
- Thank the patient at the conclusion of your examination.
- Present your positive and relevant negative findings clearly and succinctly.

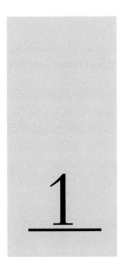

1

SCHEMES IN GENERAL SURGERY

General surgical symptoms
Examination of a lump
Examination of an ulcer
Examination of a neck lump
Examination of a thyroid lump
Examination of the breast
Examination of the chest
Examination of the abdomen
Examination of the groins
Rectal examination
General examination of the arteriopath
Examination of varicose veins

GENERAL SURGICAL SYMPTOMS

The emphasis in the short cases in the clinical section of the MRCS Examination is on clinical examination and the candidate is usually allowed to ask only a few targeted questions to the patient. The following section will help the candidate to select questions appropriate to the case he is confronted with. Note that some of the examination schemes in this book include a brief section of relevant questions that can be asked when examining a particular area.

Pain
- Site, nature, onset, duration, progression, radiation, constant/intermittent, night pain, precipitating and relieving factors, analgesia used.

Lump/ulcer
- First symptom, duration, other symptoms, progression, persistence, multiplicity (other lumps).
- Painful lump $\Rightarrow$ infection, tumour.

Cardiorespiratory symptoms
- Chest pain.
- Palpitations.
- Breathlessness.
- Cough and sputum.
- Ankle swelling.

Peripheral vascular symptoms
- Intermittent claudication (exercise tolerance: walking distance).
- Rest limb pain.
- Temperature and colour of hands and feet.

Gastrointestinal symptoms
- Appetite.
- Weight.
- Swallowing/regurgitation.
- Heartburn.
- Vomiting.

- Abdominal pain.
- Abdominal distension.
- Bowel habit.
- Flatulence.
- Jaundice.

Genitourinary symptoms:

Urinary tract symptoms
- Loin pain.
- Groin/suprapubic pain.
- Generalized oedema.
- Thirst.
- Micturition (frequency, pain, urgency, incontinence, hesitancy, terminal dribbling).
- Urine (colour, clarity, presence of blood).

Genital tract symptoms
- Menstruation.
- Pregnancies.
- Problems with sexual intercourse.
- Penile/vaginal discharge.
- Breast symptoms (pain, lumps, effect of menstrual cycle).

EXAMINATION OF A LUMP

- Introduce yourself to the patient.
- Ask the patient for permission to perform an examination.
- Expose the area to be examined adequately.
- Ask the patient if the area is painful.

Compare with other side, if possible.

Features of the lump
- Number (solitary or multiple).
- Site (measure from bony points).
- Shape.
- Size.
- Surface (smooth, irregular, rough).
- Edge (clearly defined, indistinct).
- Colour.
- Consistency (stony hard, firm, rubbery, soft, jelly-like).
- Temperature (use palmar surface of fingers).
- Tenderness.
- Relations to surrounding tissues (mobile or attached to skin, muscle or bone).

Other features
- Local tissues: skin, subcutaneous tissues, muscles, bones.
- Local blood supply and local nerve supply (sensation and muscle power).
- Regional lymph nodes. If lump is a lymph node.
- Check area drained.
- Check other lymph node groups (? generalized lymphadenopathy).
- General examination (as necessary).

Special signs
- Resonance (⇒ gas-filled).
- Fluctuation in two planes (⇒ fluid-filled).
  Paget's sign: fix small lump between two fingers and press down on lump.
- Fluid thrill (large lumps only).
- Transillumination (clear fluid: water, serum, lymph, plasma, highly refractile fat).
- Pulsatility (transmitted, expansile).
- Compressibility.
- Reducibility (⇒ hernia: check for cough impulse).
- Bruit (systolic bruit, bowel sounds).

> Note: Salivary gland lumps: remember oral examination (inspection of orifices and palpation of ducts).

Relevant questions
- Duration.
- First symptom.
- Other symptoms.
- Progression.
- Persistence.
- Multiplicity (more than one lump).
- Cause.

Examples of common lumps
Sebaceous cyst
- small firm smooth spherical swelling;
- intracutaneous (moves with skin);
- usually has a punctum;
- main sites: scalp, post-auricular area, scrotum, face (retention cyst).

Lipoma
- soft, multilobulated;
- usually subcutaneous (skin moves over it); can be subfascial or submuscular;
- no punctum;
- fluctuant.

Dermoid cyst
- firm tense cyst;
- subcutaneous;
- main sites: midline of neck, scalp, inner or outer angle of orbit.

Ganglion
- firm, tense cyst;
- subcutaneous;
- transilluminable;
- attached to a tendon or joint;
- main sites: wrist, dorsum of foot.

EXAMINATION OF AN ULCER

- Introduce yourself to the patient.
- Ask the patient for permission to perform an examination.
- Expose the area to be examined adequately.
- Ask the patient if the area is painful.

Features of the ulcer
- Site (measure from bony points).
- Shape.
- Size.
- Base (type of tissue, dead/alive, colour).
- Edge (sloping, punched out, undermined, rolled, everted).
- Depth (record in mm and anatomically – structures penetrated).
- Discharge (serous, purulent, bloody).
- Colour of surrounding skin.
- Temperature.
- Tenderness.

Other features
- Local tissues: skin, subcutaneous tissues, muscles, bones.
- Local blood supply and local nerve supply (sensation and muscle power).
- Regional lymph nodes.
- General examination (as necessary).

EXAMINATION OF A LEG ULCER

- Inspect ulcer: site, shape, size, base, edge, depth, discharge, colour of surrounding skin.
- Palpate surrounding skin: temperature, tenderness, induration.
- Palpation of peripheral pulses (and inspect for signs of poor peripheral perfusion and ausculate for arterial bruits).
- Varicose veins, signs of chronic venous insufficiency.
- Sensation.
- Adjacent joints (? neuropathic).
- Regional lymph nodes (enlarged if: 2° infection, 2° tumour deposits).
- General health of patient (e.g. cardiac failure, arrhythmias).
- Measure BP.

Relevant questions
- 'Do you smoke?'
- 'Are you diabetic?'

- 'Do you take any treatment for high blood pressure?'
- If possibly neuropathic, say 'I would like to test the patient's urine for sugar'.

Causes of leg ulcers

Venous (75%)

- supra-malleolar (gaiter area);
- 1° (due to varicose veins) or 2° (post-thrombotic);
- evidence of venous disease (varicose veins, oedema, pigmentation induration, eczema);
- good pulses.

Arterial (5%)

- shin, dorsum of foot, heel;
- no evidence of venous disease;
- no pedal pulses.

Traumatic (10%): consider neuropathy.

Miscellaneous (10%): malignancy, inflammatory bowel disease (pyoderma gangrenosum), DM, osteomyelitis, RA, Raynaud's phenomenon.

EXAMINATION OF A NECK LUMP

- Introduce yourself to the patient.
- Ask the patient for permission to perform an examination.
- Expose their neck adequately.
- Ask the patient if the area to be examined is painful.

- Identify anatomical site according to triangles of the neck (*see Diagrams 1 and 2*).

- If an obvious goitre (anterior neck lump which moves on swallowing), see **EXAMINATION OF A THYROID LUMP** (page 12).
- Assess all features of the lump (site, shape, size, surface, edge, colour, consistency, temperature, tenderness, relations to surrounding tissues, fluctuation, fluid thrill, transillumination, pulsatility, compressibility, reducibility, bruit).
- Palpate cervical lymph nodes (is lump itself a lymph node?).
- Look in mouth
  - bimanual palpation of submandibular gland or any intraoral lesion;
  - check dentition (e.g. abscesses), tongue and fauces.
- Look at scalp, ears, face.
- Listen to voice.
- Consider full ENT examination (full endoscopy of nasopharynx, larynx and hypopharynx).
- Compare with other side.
- Local tissues: skin, subcutaneous tissues, muscles, bones.
- Local blood supply and local nerve supply.
- General examination (as necessary).

CERVICAL LYMPHADENOPATHY
- Check area drained (mouth, scalp, ears, face).
- Check other lymph node groups (? generalized lymphadenopathy).
- Consider examination of breast, chest, abdomen.
- Examine for hepatosplenomegaly (reticulosis, sarcoid, glandular fever).

SALIVARY GLAND
Usually enlargement of submandibular gland or lower pole of parotid gland presents as a neck lump.
- Assess all features of the lump (site, shape, size, surface, edge, colour, consistency, temperature, tenderness, relations to surrounding tissues, fluctuation, fluid thrill, transillumination, pulsatility, compressibility, reducibility, bruit).
- Site determines whether gland is submandibular or parotid.

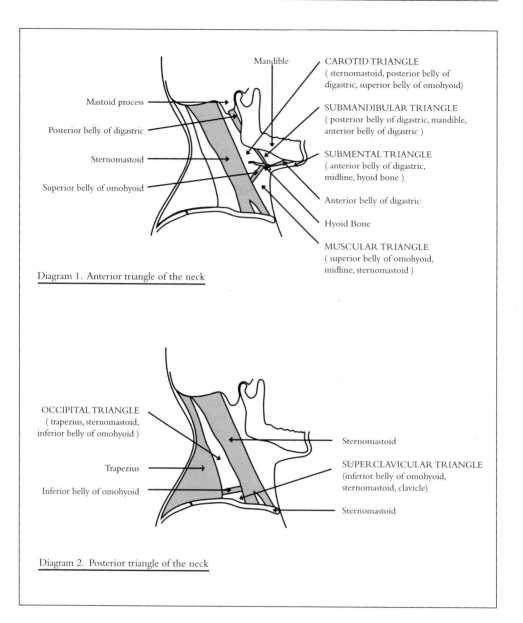

Diagram 1. Anterior triangle of the neck

Mandible

CAROTID TRIANGLE
(sternomastoid, posterior belly of
digastric, superior belly of omohyoid)

SUBMANDIBULAR TRIANGLE
(posterior belly of digastric, mandible,
anterior belly of digastric)

SUBMENTAL TRIANGLE
(anterior belly of digastric,
midline, hyoid bone)

Anterior belly of digastric

Hyoid Bone

MUSCULAR TRIANGLE
(superior belly of omohyoid,
midline, sternomastoid)

Mastoid process

Posterior belly of digastric

Sternomastoid

Superior belly of omohyoid

Diagram 2. Posterior triangle of the neck

OCCIPITAL TRIANGLE
(trapezius, sternomastoid,
inferior belly of omohyoid)

Trapezius

Inferior belly of omohyoid

Sternomastoid

SUPERCLAVICULAR TRIANGLE
(inferior belly of omohyoid,
sternomastoid, clavicle)

Sternomastoid

Submandibular gland

Examine oral cavity

- inspect duct orifice (in floor of mouth) for discharge;
- palpate duct for stones.

Bimanual palpation of gland.

Parotid gland

Examine oral cavity

- inspect duct orifice (opposite upper 2nd molar tooth) for discharge;
- palpate duct for thickening.

Examine VIIth cranial nerve

- screw up eyes;
- puff out cheeks;
- smile.

DIFFERENTIAL DIAGNOSIS OF A NECK LUMP

Lymph node

- infection
  - acute;
  - chronic.
- neoplasia
  - 1° (reticulosis);
  - 2° (metastasis).

Thyroid gland

- goitre: diffuse, multinodular, solitary nodule;
- thyroglossal cyst.

Salivary gland: tumour, stones.

Skin: sebaceous cyst, dermoid cyst, lipoma, skin tumour.

Others:

- cystic hygroma;
- branchial cyst;
- pharyngeal pouch;
- carotid body tumour, carotid aneurysm;
- subclavian aneurysm;
- sternomastoid tumour;
- cervical rib.

Cervical lymphadenopathy

Causes of lymphadenopathy

Generalized

- Infection
  - acute (e.g. glandular fever, septicaemia);
  - chronic (e.g. 2° syphilis, HIV infection).
- Neoplasia (reticulosis)
  - Hodgkin's disease;
  - non-Hodgkin's lymphoma;
  - leukaemia.
- Sarcoidosis.

Localized

Infection

- acute: dental abscess, tonsillitis;
- chronic: chronic tonsillar infection, pulmonary TB.

Metastasis

- local 1° tumour (i.e. head and neck cancer);
- distant 1° tumour: oesophagus, stomach, pancreas, breast, bronchus malignant melanoma.

Never forget general causes of lymphadenopathy

Drainage of cervical lymph nodes

Superficial cervical lymph nodes *(see Diagram 3)*

Incomplete ring around lower part of head
- Submental: tip of tongue and mental region.
- Submandibular
    - submental nodes;
    - anterior two-thirds of tongue;
    - floor of mouth (including gums and teeth);
    - nose and sinuses;
    - face;
    - anterior scalp.
- Parotid: remainder of scalp and face (including external ear).
- Mastoid: remainder of scalp and face (including external ear).
- Occipital: remainder of scalp and face (including external ear).

The superficial nodes then drain to the deep nodes.

Cervical lymph nodes (see Diagram 4)

Chain in and around carotid sheath.

Two named nodes:
- Jugulodigastric: tongue, tonsil.
- Jugulo-omohyoid: tongue.

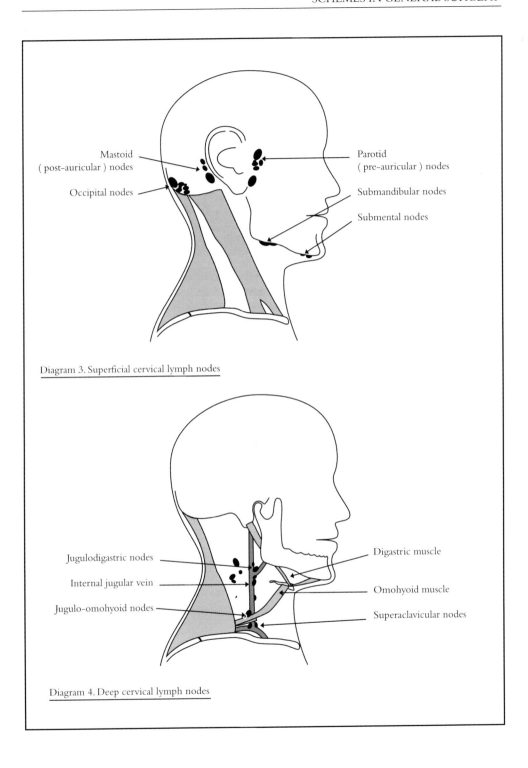

Diagram 3. Superficial cervical lymph nodes

Diagram 4. Deep cervical lymph nodes

EXAMINATION OF A THYROID LUMP

- Introduce yourself to the patient.
- Ask the patient for permission to perform an examination.
- Expose their neck adequately.

Anterior neck lump (not always midline) which moves on swallowing ⇒ thyroid lump (goitre).

Thyroid function

Perform following assessment quickly (either at beginning or end of local examination):
- Nervous/placid.
- Thin/fat.
- Under-/over-clothed.
- Myxoedematous facies.
- Thyroid eye signs
    - from side: lid retraction, exophthalmos, chemosis (oedema of conjunctiva);
    - from in front: lid retraction, exophthalmos, ophthalmoplegia, lid lag
    (see Diagram 5).
- Pretibial myxoedema.
- Pulse: rate, rhythm, volume.
- Palms: sweatiness, palmar erythema, thyroid acropathy.
- Postural tremor (outstretched arms).
- Proximal myopathy (↓ shoulder abduction ⇒ hyperthyroidism).
- Supinator reflexes (prolonged relaxation phase ⇒ hypothyroidism).

From in front
- Inspection of neck (head level and central)
    - scars;
    - neck veins;
    - lump: site, shape, size;
    - position of thyroid cartilage.
- Obvious lumps
    - ask patient to swallow (glass of water: 'Take a sip of water and hold it in your mouth until I tell you to swallow ... now swallow.')
    lump moves on swallowing ⇒ thyroid lump;
    - ask patient to open mouth and stick out tongue (ensure head kept still, e.g. by holding tongue depressor sideways between patient's clenched teeth) lump rises on tongue protrusion ⇒ thyroglossal cyst look at base of tongue (lingual thyroid).

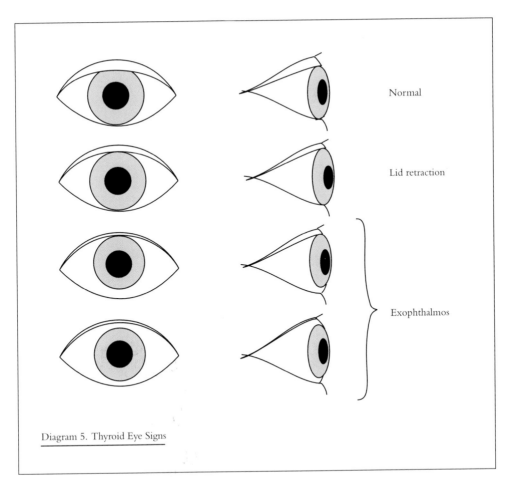

Diagram 5. Thyroid Eye Signs

- Palpate neck
    - position of trachea;
    - lump: site, shape, size, consistency (smooth, solitary nodule, multiple nodules), tenderness, mobility, movement on swallowing (keep hands still);
    - thyroglossal cyst: hold lump with one hand and place other hand on top of patient's head to steady it, then ask patient to protrude tongue.
- Palpate for retrosternal extension as thyroid falls after swallowing (one finger in suprasternal notch).
- (Percussion of retrosternal extension.)
- Listen for stridor.

From behind
- Palpate thyroid gland
    - ensure neck is relaxed.
    - palpate each lobe of thyroid in turn

- place fingers within sternomastoid muscle on both sides;
- dislocate lobe forward by gently pushing contralateral lobe backward;
- assess lump: site, shape, size, consistency (smooth, solitary nodule, multiple nodules), tenderness, mobility, movement on swallowing (keep hands still).
- Palpate carotid pulses (if pushed laterally ⇒ large benign goitre – Sir James Barrie's sign).
- Palpate cervical and supraclavicular lymph nodes.
- Auscultate for bruits (usually systolic): bell of stethoscope, patient stops breathing, occlude IJV (venous hum).

If thyroidectomy scar present, test for surgical complications:
- test for hypothyroidism; see **THYROID FUNCTION** (page 12).
- test for Chvostek's sign: gently tap over facial nerve in parotid area.
- facial muscle twitching ⇒ hypocalcaemia (due to hypoparathyroidism).
- consider testing for Trousseau's sign: inflation of sphygmomanometer cuff above diastolic BP for > 3 min.
- tetanic spasm of fingers and wrist ⇒ hypocalcaemia (due to hypoparathyroidism).
- test recurrent laryngeal nerve: ask patient to repeat a phrase ('the weather is nice today') or ask patient to cough.
- test external branch of superior laryngeal nerve: say 'eee'.

Relevant questions

Neck symptoms
- lump in neck;
- pain;
- hoarseness;
- difficulty in breathing (SOB, stridor);
- difficulty in swallowing.

Hyperthyroidism
- nervousness, irritability, insomnia, tremor;
- palpitations, SOB on exertion, ankle swelling;
- ↑ appetite, ↓ weight, ↑ bowel activity;
- preference for cold weather, sweating;
- amenorrhoea.

Eye symptoms (⇒ Graves' disease)
- staring/protruding eyes, difficulty in closing eyelids;
- double vision;
- pain.

Hypothyroidism
- ↑ weight, constipation (↓ bowel activity);
- slow thought, speech and action;
- intolerance of cold weather;
- hair loss (especially outer two-thirds eyebrow);
- muscle fatigue;
- dry skin, 'peaches and cream' complexion.

EXAMINATION OF THE BREAST

- Introduce yourself to the patient.
- Ask the patient for permission to perform an examination.
- Ask the patient to undress to the waist.
- 'Which breast is the problem?'
- 'Where in the breast is the problem?'

Inspection
- At rest (patient sitting up).
- Arms lifted up ('raise your arms up like this').
- Hands pressed on hips.

Check:
- size; symmetry/breast contour;
- skin changes (including submammary fold): puckering, *peau d'orange*, nodules, discoloration;
- ulceration, telangiectasia, surgical scars;
- nipples and areolae: inversion, discharge, skin changes;
- axillae, arms and neck.

Palpation
- Patient reclines at ~ 45°, rolled slightly to contralateral side, ipsilateral arm held relaxed above head (so breast lies flat on chest wall).
- Palpate normal breast first.
- Use flat of right hand to palpate breast circumferentially.
- Palpate
  - each quadrant;
  - areola and nipple (if history of nipple discharge, press areola circumferentially to identify duct involved);
  - axillary tail.
- Assess all features of any breast lump: site, shape, size, surface, edge, colour, consistency, temperature, tenderness, relations to surrounding tissues (mobility), fluctuation, fluid thrill.
  Test mobility of lump in two directions with pectoralis muscle both relaxed and contracted (with hands pressed on hips).

Axillae

- Support patient's elbow and forearm with your ipsilateral hand and forearm.
- Examine left axilla with right hand, examine right axilla with left hand.
- Feel systematically for palpable lymph nodes (anterior, medial, posterior and lateral walls; apex) **(see Diagram 6)**

  - pectoral nodes (drain most of breast);
  - subscapular nodes (drain axillary tail of breast);
  - central nodes;
  - lateral nodes;
  - apical nodes (drain all above nodes)

30% of normal patients have palpable axillary lymph nodes;

40% of patients with axillary lymph node metastasis have impalpable nodes.

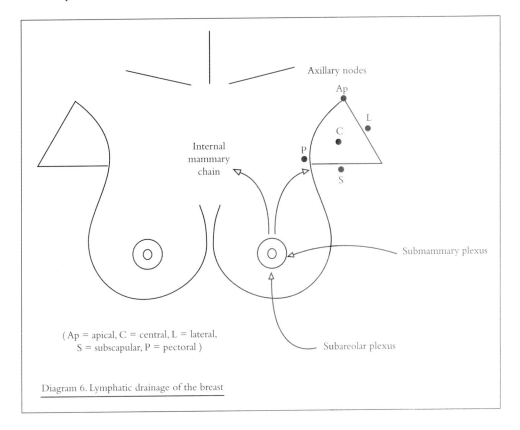

(Ap = apical, C = central, L = lateral,
S = subscapular, P = pectoral)

Diagram 6. Lymphatic drainage of the breast

General examination

- Palpate supraclavicular fossae for palpable lymph nodes.
- Examine arms for swelling (lymphoedema).
- Palpate abdomen for
  - hepatomegaly;
  - ascites;

- nodules in pouch of Douglas ('I would also like to perform a rectal examination.').
- Examine lumbar spine (percussion, movements, straight-leg raising, ankle jerks).
- Examine lung fields.

Relevant questions
- Age of patient.
- History of any lump.
- Changes during menstrual cycle.
- Menarche and menopause.
- Pregnancies and breast-feeding of any children.
- PMH.
- FH of breast/colon cancer.
- Hormonal treatment.
- Backache, headache, features of disseminated malignancy (e.g. anorexia, weight loss).

Differential diagnosis of a breast lump
- Carcinoma (always needs to excluded).
- Cyst.
- Fibroadenoma.
- Others (5%)
    - traumatic: fat necrosis;
    - other cysts: galactocoele, chronic abscess, cystadenoma, retention cyst;
    - other tumours: duct papilloma, sarcoma;
    - chest wall swellings: rib tumour, TB, lipoma, eroding aortic aneurysm, Mondor's disease (superficial vein thrombosis).

Clinical features of common breast lumps:
- Irregular and indistinct
    - hard: carcinoma;
    - rubbery: fibroadenosis.

- Smooth and distinct
    - hard: cyst (fibroadenosis);
    - rubbery: fibroadenoma.

EXAMINATION OF THE CHEST

Essentially, examination of the chest wall and respiratory system.
Examination of the cardiovascular system: see **GENERAL EXAMINATION OF THE ARTERIOPATH** (page 34).

- Introduce yourself to the patient.
- Ask the patient for permission to perform an examination.
- Position the patient erect (sitting or standing).
- Expose their chest completely.
- Unless necessary, be discrete in exposing external genitalia (consider a patient's privacy in the examination setting).
- Observe general appearance: cyanosis, shortness of breath, cachexia.
- Listen to the patient's voice when answering questions: hoarseness.

General examination
- Examine hands: clubbing, peripheral cyanosis, tobacco staining.
- Palpate radial pulse: bounding pulse $\Rightarrow CO_2$ retention.
- Glance at eyes: pupils (Horner's syndrome), conjunctivae (anaemia, polycythaemia).
- Inspect tongue (cyanosis).
- Observe height of JVP.
- Palpate cervical and supraclavicular lymph nodes.

Examine anterior chest then posterior chest (patient sitting forward).

Inspection
- Chest wall: shape, scars, lumps.
- Chest movements (from end of bed while patient takes deep breath): symmetry, expansion, use of accessory muscles in neck.
- Respiratory rate (crude rate = number of inspirations in 15 seconds $\times$ 4).
- Respiratory pattern.
- If a mass is found: determine its characteristics (site, shape, size, surface, edge, consistency, tenderness, relations, resonance, fluctuation, pulsatility, bruit).

Palpation
- Trachea in suprasternal notch (with head partially extended): check trachea is central. Deviation $\Rightarrow$ fibrosis, collapse of upper lobe or whole lung, pneumothorax, very large pleural effusion (non-chest causes: goitre, spinal asymmetry).
- Apex beat: lateral displacement $\Rightarrow$ mediastinal shift.

- Chest expansion while patient takes deep breath (feel both sides for symmetry): diminished movement ⇒ pathology on same side.
- Tactile vocal fremitus (ask patient to say 'ninety-nine'): ↑ over areas of consolidation.
- Axillary lymph nodes.

Percussion
- Percuss down both sides (including clavicles)
    - dullness ⇒ pleural thickening, collapse, consolidation, fibrosis (upper lobe fibrosis ⇒ old TB);
    - stony dullness ⇒ pleural effusion;
    - resonance and diminished movement ⇒ pneumothorax, large bulla.

Auscultation
- Breath sounds: ↓ breath sounds ⇒ effusion, pleural thickening, pneumothorax airway obstruction.
- Length of inspiration (*I*) and expiration (*E*)
    - normal: $I > E$;
    - bronchial breathing: $I = E$;
    - obstructive airways disease: $E > I$.
- Added sounds
    - wheeze ⇒ asthma, bronchitis, LVF;
    - fine crackles ⇒ LVF, fibrosing alveolitis;
    - coarse crackles ⇒ excess bronchial secretions;
    - friction rub ⇒ pleurisy.
- Vocal resonance (ask patient to say 'ninety-nine'): ↑ over areas of consolidation (whispering pectoriloquy also may be present).

- To examiner: 'I would also like to examine the patient's sputum'.

Common causes of chest signs
- Clubbing
    - Ca bronchus, empyema, lung abscess, fibrosing alveolitis;
    - cyanotic congenital heart disease, subacute bacterial endocarditis;
    - Crohn's disease, ulcerative colitis, cirrhosis.
(**See table opposite**)

X-ray
- Erect PA: standard projection.
- AP (sitting or supine): seriously ill patients.

	Movements on side of lesion	Trachea	Percussion	Breath sounds	Tactile fremitus vocal resonance
Pleural effusion	↓	Central (away from large effusion)	Stony dull	↓ and bronchial breathing at top of effusion	↓
Pneumothorax	↓	Central (away from large pneumothorax)	Hyperresonant	↓	↓
Consolidation (pneumonia)	↓	Central (towards consolidation if collapse)	Dull	Bronchial (absent if airway obstructed)	↑ (↓if airway obstructed)
Fibrosis	↓	Towards upper lobe fibrosis	Dull	Bronchial	↑
Chronic obstructive pulmonary disease	↓	Central ± tug	Normal or hyperresonant	Scattered added sounds	Normal

- Potential pitfalls
    - AP film: cardiomegaly, wide mediastinum, high diaphragm, vague lower zone shadowing, rotation artefacts;
    - supine film: small pneumothorax missed, pleural effusion appears as diffuse shadowing.

Additional views
- Lateral: identification of abnormalities seen on PA/AP view (e.g. foreign body).
- Lateral decubitus (abnormal side down): small pleural effusion, subpulmonary pneumothorax.

- Sternal view: suspected fractured sternum.
- Rib views: rarely indicated (rib fractures diagnosed clinically).
- Expiration films: small pneumothorax.

Alternative imaging
- US
- CT
- MRI

Assessment of PA chest radiograph
- Adequacy
    - projection and exposure (intervertebral discs clearly visible);
    - posture (supine or erect);
    - rotation (spinous processes central relative to medial ends of clavicles);
    - degree of inspiration (right hemidiaphragm: anterior end R6/7 or posterior end R9).
- Alignment: thoracic spine.
- Position of any invasive equipment (e.g. ETT, central venous cannula).
- Mediastinum
    - upper mediastinum (width, aortic outline, double outline $\Rightarrow$ pneumomediastinum);
    - hila;
    - size and shape of heart.
- Diaphragm: cardiophrenic and costophrenic angles.
- Lung fields: fissures, opacities (remember apices).
- Bones
    - ribs;
    - clavicles;
    - scapulae;
    - shoulder joints;
    - thoracic spine.
- Extrathoracic
    - soft tissues;
    - surgical emphysema;
    - breast shadows;
    - free gas under diaphragm (pneumoperitoneum).

EXAMINATION OF THE ABDOMEN

- Introduce yourself to the patient.
- Ask the patient for permission to perform an examination.
- Position the patient supine with one pillow.
- Expose their abdomen completely.
- Unless necessary, be discrete in exposing external genitalia (consider a patient's privacy in the examination setting).
- Ask the patient if their abdomen is painful.

General examination
- Inspect hands: clubbing, koilonychia, Dupuytren's contracture, palmar erythema, spider naevi.
- Flapping tremor: if hepatic encephalopathy suspected.
- Eyes: jaundice (sclerae), anaemia (conjunctivae).
- Inspect tongue (ulcers).
- Look for spider naevi on face and chest.
- Palpate cervical and supraclavicular (especially left) lymph nodes.

Inspection
- Stand at end of bed.
- Observe abdomen while patient takes deep breath for
    - cachexia;
    - asymmetry;
    - general distension ($\pm$ eversion of umbilicus);
    - localized mass;
    - visible epigastric pulsation;
    - visible peristalsis;
    - distended veins (in portal hypertension, IVC obstruction);
    - scars, striae, rashes;
    - pigmentation;
    - hair distribution;
    - hernial sites (ask patient to lift his head against resistance).

Palpation
- Kneel on floor or sit so that eyes are ~50 cm above patient and examining arm is horizontal.
- (Examine external genitalia first, if appropriate.)

- Ask patient if there is any localized abdominal tenderness.
- Light palpation for tenderness and masses/organomegaly (ask patient if there is any painful area and start in quadrant away from any area of pain/if no pain start in RUQ).
- Look at patient's face while palpating.
- Deeper palpation.
- If a mass is found determine its characteristics (site, shape, size, surface, edge, consistency, tenderness, relations, resonance, fluctuation, pulsatility, bruit).
- Palpate for liver, starting from RIF: percuss out upper (N: 4th/5th intercostal space) and lower borders. If enlarged auscultate for bruit.
- Palpate for spleen, starting from RIF (if difficult ask patient to roll onto right side): distinct lower edge, cannot get above it, medial notch, dull to percussion along 10th rib.
- Palpate for kidneys: ballottable between hand in front and hand in loin (retroperitoneal masses may be more easily felt with patient in knee–elbow position).
- Palpate for abdominal aortic aneurysm (hand flat in epigastrium – Fox's manoeuvre).
- Palpate groins for inguinal lymph nodes.
- Check hernial orifices (two femoral, two inguinal, one umbilical).

Percusion
- Percussion
- Ascites
    - shifting dullness (if dull in flanks)
        - central resonance and flank dullness when supine;
        - central dullness and flank resonance when lateral.
    - fluid thrill (if large effusion suspected): thrill felt on opposite flank when one flank 'flicked'.

Auscultation
- Bruits (especially renal artery stenosis).
- Bowel sounds.

- To examiner: 'I would also like to examine the patient's genitalia and perform a rectal examination'.

Common causes of abdominal signs
- *Clubbing*: cirrhosis, inflammatory bowel disease, many non–abdominal causes.
- *Palmar erythema*: chronic liver disease, RA, pregnancy, leukaemia, hyperthyroidism.
- *Hepatomegaly*: right heart failure, early cirrhosis, metastases, infective hepatitis.

- *Splenomegaly*: myelofibrosis, leukaemia (chronic myeloid > chronic lymphatic), lymphoma, haemolytic anaemias, portal hypertension, infections.
- *Ascites*: portal hypertension (cirrhosis, metastases, Budd–Chiari), hypoproteinaemia (renal disease, cirrhosis, cachexia, enteropathies), chronic peritonitis (TB, secondary deposits), chylous ascites.

Causes of abdominal masses

Some are unlikely to be encountered in the examination setting.
- RUQ: hepatomegaly, Riedel's lobe, enlarged gall bladder.
- Epigastrium: stomach tumour, transverse colon tumour, enlarged para-aortic lymph nodes.
- LUQ: splenomegaly, stomach tumour, splenic flexure tumour.

- Loins/flanks: renal tumour.
- Central: large/small bowel mass, retroperitoneal mass (lymph nodes, pancreatic tumour, abdominal aortic aneurysm), herniae.

- RIF: Ca caecum, Crohn's disease, appendix abscess, ileocaecal TB, actinomycosis, intussusception).
- LIF: Ca sigmoid colon, diverticular disease.
- RIF or LIF: ovarian mass, ectopic kidney, transplanted kidney, psoas abscess, iliac artery aneurysm.
- Suprapubic: retention of urine, bladder tumour, pregnancy, fibroids, uterine tumour.

X-ray

- Supine abdomen: standard projection.
- Erect chest: most sensitive radiograph for detecting small pneumoperitoneum.

Additional views
- Erect abdomen: rarely required to show air–fluid levels.
- Left lateral decubitus: alternative to erect abdominal radiograph if patient cannot sit or stand.

Alternative imaging
- US
- CT
- MRI

Assessment of supine abdominal radiograph

Difficult to interpret because it is asymmetrical and has great individual variability in normal appearances.

- Adequacy
- Alignment: lumbar spine
- Bones
    - lower ribs;
    - lumbar transverse processes;
    - sacrum/pelvis;
    - femoral head/neck;
    - fractures suggest possible underlying soft tissue injury (e.g. liver, spleen, kidney).
- Cartilage and joints (joint space)
    - sacroiliac joints;
    - pubic symphysis;
    - hip joints.
- Soft tissues
    - bowel gas pattern (maximum diameters: small bowel 2.5 cm, large bowel 5.5 cm);
    - free air (pneumoperitoneum);
    - air in biliary tree or portal vein;
    - size of organs;
    - fat–tissue interfaces;
    - abnormal calcification.

Assessment of erect chest radiograph

- Adequacy
    - mid-thoracic intervertebral discs clearly visible;
    - spinous processes central relative to medial ends of clavicles.
- Position of invasive equipment (e.g. ETTs, central venous cannulae).
- Mediastinum
    - upper mediastinum (width, aortic outline, double outline $\Rightarrow$ pneumo-mediastinum);
    - hila;
    - size and shape of heart.
- Diaphragm: cardiophrenic and costophrenic angles.
- Lung fields: fissures, opacities (remember apices).
- Bones
    - ribs;
    - clavicles;
    - scapulae;
    - shoulder joints;
    - thoracic spine.

- Extrathoracic soft tissues
  - surgical emphysema;
  - breast shadows;
  - free gas under diaphragm (pneumoperitoneum).

EXAMINATION OF THE GROINS

Hernia
- Protusion of a viscus (or part of a viscus) through its coverings into abdomal position.
- Usually a diverticulum of the peritoneal cavity.
- Components: sac (peritoneum) and coverings and contents.

- Introduce yourself to the patient.
- Ask the patient for permission to perform an examination.
- Ask the patient to stand up.
- Expose their groins.
- Ask the patient if the area is painful.
- 'Do you have a lump? Can you show me where it is?'

- Inspect both sides from in front.
- Look for: scars of previous surgery, any obvious lumps.
- Examine scrotum from in front; see **EXAMINATION OF A SCROTAL SWELLING** (page 30).
- Palpate any inguinal lump from the side: site, shape, size, surface, edge, consistency, temperature, tenderness, fluctuation, pulsatility, reducibility.
- Compress lump, ask patient to turn head away and cough: expansile cough impulse ⇒ hernia.

- Ask the patient to lie down.
- 'Can you put the lump back yourself?'
- If not, attempt to reduce lump
     - reducibility ⇒ hernia (or saphena varix);
     - direct inguinal hernia: may be able to feel defect in abdominal wall;
     - inguinal hernia: arises above and lateral but bulges medial to pubic tubercle;
     - femoral hernia
          - arises below and lateral to pubic tubercle;
          - tends to extend lower down;
          - tends to push up groin crease.
- Place two fingers over deep inguinal ring (1 cm above midpoint of inguinal ligament).
- Ask the patient to stand up.
- Ask patient to turn head away and cough: control ⇒ indirect inguinal hernia.

- Inspect legs for varicose veins ($\Rightarrow$ saphena varix).
- Examine other side.
- Examine abdomen.
- 'I would also like to perform a rectal examination.'
- 'May I wash my hands, please?'

Note: Some examiners advocate supine examination first.

Relevant questions
- Occupation (relevant to aetiology and management).
- Cough.
- Constipation (and consider large bowel malignancy).
- Straining at micturition.

Differential diagnosis of a groin swelling
- Inguinal hernia (direct/indirect).
- Femoral hernia.
- Incisional hernia.
- Saphena varix.
- Femoral artery aneurysm.
- Lymphadenopathy (e.g. enlarged lymph node of Cloquet).
- Psoas abscess.
- Ectopic testis.
- Hydrocoele of cord (males) or hydrocoele of canal of Nuck (females).
- Bartholin's cyst (females).
- Skin lump.

Diagnosis	Structure involved	Relation to inguinal ligament
Lipoma, fibroma, haemangioma	Skin/subcutaneous tissues	Either
Saphena varix	Femoral vein	Below
Femoral artery aneurysm	Femoral artery	Below
Lymphadenopathy	Inguinal/femoral lymph nodes	Either
Psoas abscess	Psoas sheath	Below
Hydrocoele of cord, ectopic testis	Testicular apparatus	Above
Inguina hernia (indirect/direct)	Hernial orifices	Above
Femoral hernia		Below

Examination of a scrotal swelling

- Inspect all of scrotal skin (front and back).
- Inspect scrotal contents: site, shape, asymmetry.
- Palpate scrotal contents using both hands: testis, epididymis, cord.
- Examine any swelling
    - general characteristics (site, shape, size, surface, edge, consistency, temperature);
    - can you get above swelling? If not ⇒ inguino-scrotal hernia;
    - can you define testis and epididymis?;
    - does swelling transilluminate?;
    - tenderness?;
    - expansile cough impulse?
- Examine perineum.
- Examine for inguinal lymph nodes.
- 'I would also like to perform a rectal examination.'

Differential diagnosis of a scrotal swelling (*see Diagram 7*)

- Indirect inguinal hernia.
- Hydrocoele.
- Hydrocoele of the cord.
- Haematocoele.
- Varicocoele.
- Spermatocoele.
- Epididymal cyst.
- Epididymo-orchitis (acute).
- Acute epididymitis.
- Acute orchitis.
- Chronic epididymitis.
- Gumma (syphilis).
- TB.
- Testicular tumour.
- Torsion of testis.

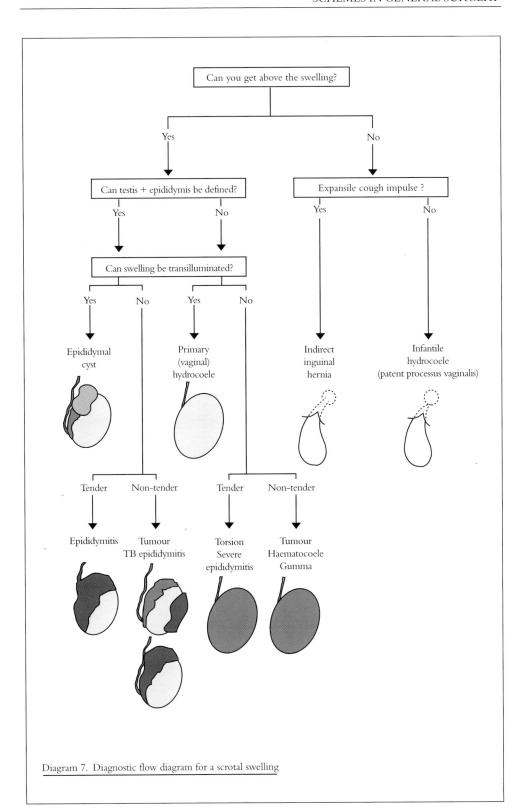

Diagram 7. Diagnostic flow diagram for a scrotal swelling

RECTAL EXAMINATION

Fistula
- Abnormal connection between two epothelial-lined surfaces.

Sinus
- Abnormal track lined by epithelial cells, communicating with a lumen or hollow viscus.

- Not required in the examination setting.

- Introduce yourself to the patient.
- Ask the patient for permission to perform an examination.
- Be considerate of the patient's embarrassment.
- Ask the patient to lie in left lateral position with knees raised to chest.
- Expose anus using left hand.
- Perform digital rectal examination using gloved right index finger.

Inspection
- External haemorrhoids.
- Fistulae/sinuses/fissures.
- Anal masses.
- Skin excoriation.
- Sentinel pile.
- Ulcers.
- Warts.
- Perianal soiling.
- Blood/mucus.
- No anus.

Palpation
- Anal tone (ask patient to bear down – perineal descent, puborectalis 'shrug', incontinence).
- Masses: site, size, shape, fixity, induration.
- Prostate.
- Faecal consistency.
- Tenderness.

Differential diagnosis of a rectal mass

Lumen:

- faeces.

Wall:

- Ca rectum/anal canal;
- benign tumour of rectum/anal canal (polyp);
- amoebic granuloma;
- intersphincteric abscess.

Pouch of Douglas:

- Ca sigmoid colon;
- diverticular disease;
- pelvic abscess;
- peritoneal deposits → 'frozen pelvis';
- endometriosis.

Outside wall:

- mesorectal lymphadenopathy;
- enlarged prostate (benign prostatic hyperplasia, Ca);
- cervical tumour;
- uterine tumour;
- ovarian tumour.

GENERAL EXAMINATION OF THE ARTERIOPATH

- Introduce yourself to the patient.
- Ask the patient for permission to perform an examination.

- Note whether patient can lie flat during the examination (? orthopnoea).
- Inspect skin (fingertips, palmar creases, lips) and mucous membranes (conjunctivae): anaemia, polycythaemia, cyanosis.
- Note any nicotine-staining of fingers.
- Palpate upper limb pulses (both sides simultaneously): radial artery, brachial artery.
- Note radial pulse characteristics: rate, rhythm, strength, nature of pulse wave (normal, flattened or anacrotic, accentuated or 'water-hammer').
- Measure BP in both arms.
- Palpate carotid pulse (rate, rhythm, character, volume, state of vessel wall).
- Auscultate for arterial bruits: carotid, subclavian (supraclavicular fossa).
- Observe JVP (height from sternal angle, wave form).

- Palpate apex for position, heaves and thrills.
- Auscultate for heart murmurs
    - apex (45° erect and left lateral position);
    - below sternum;
    - 2nd right intercostal space (45° erect and sitting forwards);
    - left sternal edge (45° erect and sitting forwards).
- Auscultate lung bases posteriorly.

- Palpate abdomen for abdominal aortic aneurysm.
- Auscultate for arterial bruits: renal (epigastrium or posteriorly in loins), mesenteric (epigastrium).
- Inspect for sacral and ankle oedema.

Lower limbs (*see Diagram 8*)

Inspection
- Skin colour.
- Hair loss, ulcers, amputations (e.g. of toes).
- Buerger's test (for severe ischaemia)
    - foot becomes pale on elevation of leg;
    - foot becomes markedly red when dependent (reactive hyperaemia);
    - Buerger's angle (angle of raised leg $\Rightarrow$ pallor): $< 20°$ $\Rightarrow$ severe ischaemia.

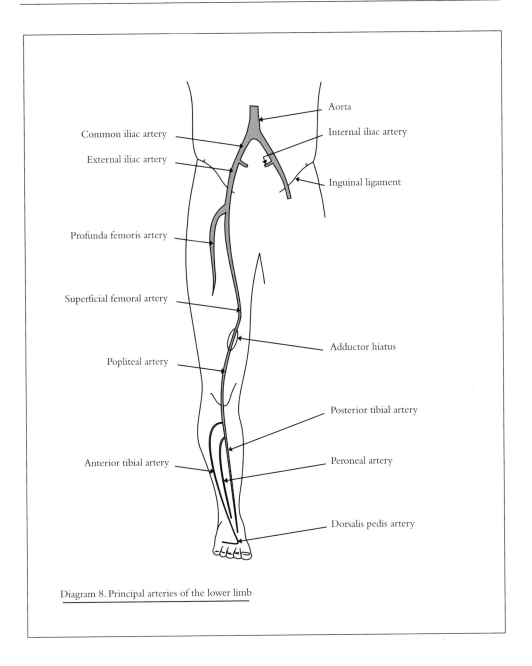

Diagram 8. Principal arteries of the lower limb

- Capillary filling time (time for blanched nail bed to become pink again).
- Venous filling/guttering.
- Ischaemic changes: pressure areas (heel, malleoli, head of 5th metatarsal, under head of 1st metatarsal, tips of toes, between toes).
- Signs of arterial embolism.

Palpation

- Temperature.
- Lower limb pulses: femoral, popliteal, posterior tibial and dorsalis pedis
    - absent femoral pulses ⇒ aortoiliac disease;
    - normal femoral but absent foot pulses ⇒ femorodistal disease;
    - normal pulses at rest disappear or weaken on exercise;
    - normal pulses at rest unaffected by exercise.

Auscultation

- Femoral bruits.

Relevant questions

Assessment of risk factors

- Smoking.
- ↑ BP.
- DM.
- History of CVA/TIA.
- History of MI/ischaemic heart disease.
- Family history of significant arterial disease < 60 years old.

Assessment of leg ischaemia

Classification

- Acute.
- Chronic
    - intermittent claudication: muscular pain only on exercise and relieved by rest due to mild ischaemia;
    - rest pain: pain in affected foot at rest, becoming intolerable due to severe ischaemia;
    - critical ischaemia: persistently recurring rest pain requiring regular analgesia *or* ulceration or gangrene of foot or toes; arterial insufficiency severe enough to threaten viability of foot.

Clinical features

- Pain.
- Paraesthesia.
- Paralysis.
- Pallor.
- Pulseless.
- (Perishingly) cold.

Asymmetrical loss of pulses (normal contralateral limb) ⇒ embolism.
Symmetrical loss of pulses ⇒ thrombosis.

Further investigations
- Hand–held Doppler ultrasound probe
  - presence/absence of pulses;
  - ankle systolic blood pressure;
  - ankle/brachial pressure index (ABPI): at rest and after exercise.
- Duplex Doppler scan.
- Arteriography.

Causes of leg pain on walking
- Vascular claudication.
- Arthritis (e.g. of hip, knee, ankle, subtalar joint).
- Spinal claudication (spinal stenosis).
- Sciatica (intervertebral disc prolapse).
- Venous insufficiency.

EXAMINATION OF VARICOSE VEINS

Anatomy (*see Diagrams 9 and 10*)
- Long saphenous vein (LSV) passes in front of medial malleolus, runs up medial aspect of leg and thigh, and drains into femoral vein at saphenofemoral junction (SFJ).
- SFJ lies two fingerbreadths below and lateral to pubic tubercle.
- Short saphenous vein (SSV) passes behind lateral malleolus and drains into popliteal vein in popliteal fossa, or occasionally into LSV more proximally.
- 90% of varicose veins involve the long saphenous vein (LSV).

- Introduce yourself to the patient.
- Ask the patient for permission to perform an examination.
- Ask the patient to stand up.
- Expose the lower limbs up to the groins but be discrete and do not expose external genitalia.

Inspection
- Distribution: long or short saphenous vein
  - above knee varicosities $\Rightarrow$ saphenofemoral incompetence, involving LSV;
  - posterolateral calf varicosities feeding into popliteal fossa $\Rightarrow$ short saphenous vein (SSV) involved.
- Severity of varicose veins (exclude spider veins), e.g. corona phlebectasia.
- Skin changes ($\Rightarrow$ chronic venous insufficiency): swelling, lipodermatosclerosis, eczema, ulcers.

Palpation
- Peripheral pulses (to exclude arterial disease).
- Groin (? saphena varix).
- Cough impulse (bulge and thrill palpable at SFJ).
- Palpation of individual varicosities.

Percussion
Tap test (+ve if tapping a large varicosity produces a palpable impulse at SFJ).

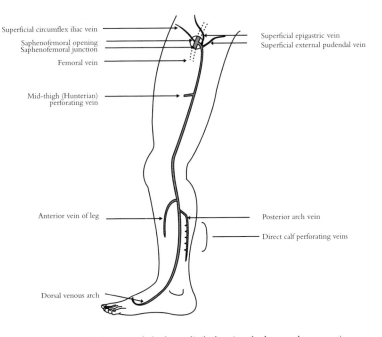

Superficial circumflex iliac vein

Saphenofemoral opening
Saphenofemoral junction

Femoral vein

Mid-thigh (Hunterian)
perforating vein

Superficial epigastric vein
Superficial external pudendal vein

Anterior vein of leg

Posterior arch vein

Direct calf perforating veins

Dorsal venous arch

Diagram 9. Medial aspect of the lower limb showing the long saphenous vein

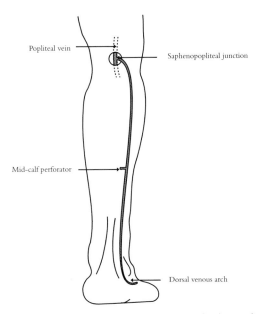

Popliteal vein

Saphenopopliteal junction

Mid-calf perforator

Dorsal venous arch

Diagram 10. Posterior aspect of the leg showing the short saphenous vein

Special tests

Trendelenburg test
- lie patient down, elevate limb and massage proximally to empty veins;
- place hand over SFJ and apply gentle pressure;
- ask patient to stand up;
- observe any filling of varicosities;
- +ve if varicosities controlled ($\Rightarrow$ saphenofemoral incompetence).

Tourniquet test (or timed tourniquet test)
- as for Trendelenburg test but using tourniquet at different levels;
- control at upper thigh $\Rightarrow$ saphenofemoral incompetence;
- control above knee $\Rightarrow$ mid-thigh perforator incompetence;
- control below knee $\Rightarrow$ short saphenopopliteal incompetence;
- no control $\Rightarrow$ distal perforator incompetence.

Perthe's test (test of perforator incompetence): as for Trendelenburg test but using high thigh tourniquet and calf exercise.

Examination of abdomen and pelvis

Investigations
- Hand-held Doppler: reflux signal at SFJ $\Rightarrow$ aphenofemoral incompetence.
- Duplex Doppler.
- Varicography.

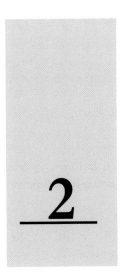

2

SCHEMES IN ORTHOPAEDICS

Orthopaedic symptoms
Examination of a joint
Examination of the shoulder
Examination of the elbow
Examination of the wrist
Examination of the hand
Examination of the hip
Examination of the knee
Examination of the ankle and foot
Examination of the cervical spine
Examination of the thoracolumbar spine
Examination of the peripheral nervous system
Examination of the brachial plexus
Examination of the peripheral nerve lesions
Examination of a multiple trauma patient

ORTHOPAEDIC SYMPTOMS

- Pain.
- Stiffness.
- Swelling.
- Deformity.
- Change in sensation.
- Loss of function.

Pain
Commonest symptom.

> **Note**: Site, duration, onset, radiation, constant/intermittent, night pain, precipitating and relieving factors, analgesia used.

Sources
- joint;
- bone;
- soft tissues (muscle, tendon, ligament, capsule, bursa);
- referred.

Stiffness
- Limited movement.
- ± Locking
    - a sudden inability to complete a certain movement;
    - suggests a mechanical block (e.g. loose body, flap tear of a meniscus).

Swelling
- Can arise from soft tissues, joint, bone.
- Constant/intermittent.
- Pain $\Rightarrow$ infection, tumour.
- Rate of joint swelling:
    - rapid $\Rightarrow$ haemarthrosis;
    - slower $\Rightarrow$ effusion.

Deformity
- Shortening/lengthening.
- Malalignment.

Change in sensation
- Paraesthesia/numbness ⇒ interference with nerve function.
- Causes
    - pressure from a neighbouring structure (e.g. prolapsed disc);
    - local ischaemia (e.g. nerve entrapment in a fibro-osseous tunnel);
    - peripheral neuropathy.

Loss of function
- More than one joint may contribute to disability.
- Lower limb
    - exercise tolerance (walking distance);
    - exercise limiting factor (consider cardiovascular and peripheral vascular causes);
    - mobility aids used: sticks, crutches, frame;
    - ability to use stairs, ability to get from a chair to standing;
    - ability with shoes, socks, toenail cutting (pedicure).
- Upper limb
    - hand dominance;
    - ability with feeding, personal hygiene, brushing hair, writing, etc.
- Occupation.
- Home circumstances: type of accommodation, stairs, cohabitants/warden, social services.

EXAMINATION OF A JOINT

- Look.
- Feel.
- Move.
- X-ray.

- Introduce yourself to the patient.
- Ask the patient for permission to perform an examination.
- Expose the joint to be examined adequately, together with the 'normal' side for comparison.
- Do not expose external genitalia (consider a patient's privacy in the examination setting).
- Ask the patient if the joint is painful.

Look
- General attitude/appearance.
- Posture.
- Gait
    - normal gait cycle: stance phase (heel strike → foot flat → toe off) → swing phase;
    - abnormal gait = a limp.
- Skin: discoloration, wounds, scars, abnormal creases, sinuses, callosities.
- Shape
    - swelling, wasting (measure using a tape measure), lumps;
    - deformity (postural, fixed).
- Position: attitude of limb.
- Compare with the opposite limb (record pattern of joint involvement if polyarticular).
- Measure (if appropriate): e.g. limb length (apparent and true).

Feel
Note any tenderness (look at patient's expression).
- Skin: temperature, moisture, sensation (light touch, pinprick, two-point discrimination).
- Soft tissues: lumps (site, size, shape, surface, surroundings, consistency, transilluminability), thickening, wasting.
- Bones and joints: outlines, synovial thickening, effusion (fluid swelling).

Move
Active

- range of movement (see below);
- power (movement against resistance and palpate muscle belly for contraction).

Passive

- range of movement (see below);
- abnormal movements (joint instability, movement at a fracture site).

Note: Pain and position of comfort (look at patient's expression)
Crepitus

Movements to test

- Flexion/extension.
- Abduction/adduction.
- Internal/external rotation.
- (Lateral flexion).
- (Lateral rotation).
- (Pronation/supination).
- (Circumduction).
- (Inversion/eversion).
- (Opposition).

Range of joint movement

- Varies among individuals.
- Depends on age, gender, race and even occupation.
- Slightly greater in children than in adults.
- Decreases with age, but this loss is relatively small in most normal joints.
- Measured using a goniometer (joint protractor) $\Rightarrow$ more accurate than visual estimation.
- Zero starting position: extended 'anatomical position' of the extremity.
- Compare with opposite side (wherever possible).
- Throughout this book, the average range of joint movement for a young adult is recorded in brackets after the movement, e.g. flexion (160°).

Evidence of generalized ligamentous laxity (Beighton's 9 – point test)
One point for each side
- Thumb can reach forearm.
- 90° extension of little finger MCPJ.
- Elbow hyperextension >10°.
- Knee hyperextension >10°.
- Thoracolumbar forward flexion such that palms lie flat on floor.

Neurological examination

Peripheral vascular examination (including peripheral pulses)

X-ray
An X-ray film is strictly termed a radiograph.

Consider the following when requesting skeletal radiographs
- Two views: usually AP and lateral.
- Two joints: above and below area of interest.
- Two sides: comparison views are especially useful in children (epiphyses can cause difficulties in interpretation).
- Two occasions: e.g. developing disease, monitoring of healing.

Assessment of a joint radiograph (ABCS system)
- Adequacy (and quality).
- Alignment (of bones).
- Bones (margins, density, continuity of trabecular pattern).
- Cartilage and joints (joint space).
- Soft tissues.

Alternative imaging modalities
- Tomography.
- Arthrography.
- Myelography/discography.
- CT.
- MRI.
- Ultrasound.
- Radioisotope bone scan.
- Bone densitometry.

EXAMINATION OF THE SHOULDER

Anatomy

The shoulder girdle is a complex composed of five joints:

- Glenohumeral joint (the 'shoulder joint');
- Scapulothoracic articulation;
- Coracoacromial arch (subacromial joint);
- Acromioclavicular joint (ACJ);
- Sternoclavicular joint (SCJ);

- Introduce yourself to the patient.
- Ask the patient for permission to perform an examination.
- Adequately expose both upper limbs.
- Ask patient if their shoulder is painful.

Consider examination of the cervical spine in a case of shoulder pain.

Look (from in front and from behind).

- Skin: scars, sinuses.
- Shape: look for shoulder asymmetry.

  From behind
  - contour of shoulder;
  - wasting of deltoid/supraspinatus/infraspinatus;
  - shape of scapula, winging of scapula.

  From in front
  - contour of shoulder;
  - wasting of pectoral muscles;
  - anterior glenohumeral dislocation;
  - joint swelling;
  - prominent ACJ (subluxation, OA);
  - deformity of clavicle (old fracture);
  - prominent SCJ (subluxation).
- Position: e.g. internal rotation $\Rightarrow$ posterior dislocation.

Feel (from behind or alongside patient).
Note any tenderness.

- (Skin: temperature.)

- Soft tissues
- tendons
    - supraspinatus: internally rotate shoulder and palpate just anterior to acromion;
    - long head of biceps: palpate anteriorly in bicipital groove as shoulder is internally and externally rotated.
    - ligaments (coracoacromial, coracoclavicular);
    - trapezius (spasm ⇒ neck problem).
- Bones and joints
    - coracoid;
    - glenohumeral joint;
    - humeral head (direct and via axilla);
    - greater tuberosity (anterolateral to outer border of acromion);
    - acromion;
    - ACJ;
    - clavicle;
    - SCJ.

Move

Normal range of movement *(see Diagram 11)*. Note that the scapular plane is 30° anterior to the coronal plane.

Active (patient asked to imitate examiner).
- Abduction ('lift both arms up to the side'): assess range, rhythm and pain *(see Diagram 12)*
    - scapulothoracic movement normally starts at 30-40° abduction;
    - normal scapulohumeral rhythm: glenohumeral/scapulothoracic ratio = 2:1;
    - difficult initiation/humeral head rises up ⇒ rotator cuff tear;
    - low painful arc (60-120°) ⇒ subacromial (rotator cuff) pathology
    - high painful arc (140-180°) ⇒ OA ACJ;
    - if a painful arc is present, repeat abduction with palpation under acromion: ↑ pain confirms subacromial pathology.

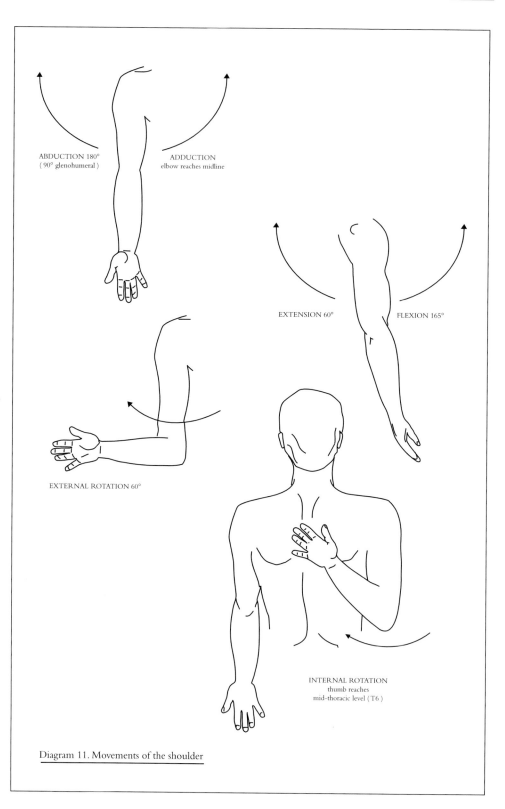

ABDUCTION 180°
(90° glenohumeral)

ADDUCTION
elbow reaches midline

EXTENSION 60°

FLEXION 165°

EXTERNAL ROTATION 60°

INTERNAL ROTATION
thumb reaches
mid-thoracic level (T6)

Diagram 11. Movements of the shoulder

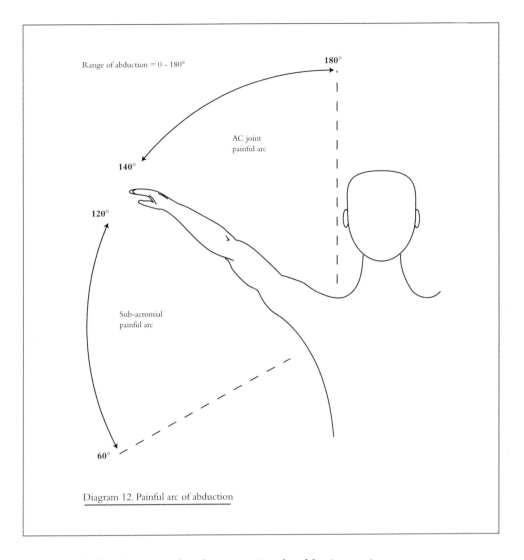

Diagram 12. Painful arc of abduction

- Adduction (each hand to opposite shoulder in turn);
- Flexion (forward elevation) ('lift both arms forwards'): compensatory lumbar spine extension can be eliminated by examination supine;
- Extension ('lift both arms backwards');
- External rotation in abduction (hands behind head);
- Internal rotation in adduction (hands behind back);
- Circumduction.

Passive

- Abduction (180°, 90° glenohumeral): press down on acromion or fix inferior pole of scapula to eliminate scapulothoracic movement;
- (Adduction: elbow reaches midline);
- Flexion (165°);
- Extension (60°);
- External rotation (arms held to side with elbow flexed 90°) (60°): movement most affected in frozen shoulder;
- Internal rotation in extension/posterior reach (measure level thumb tip can reach up back) (mid-thoracic level [T6] or medial border of opposite scapula): requires shoulder extension and elbow flexion;
- External rotation in abduction (abducted 90° and elbow flexed 90°) (100°)
- Internal rotation in abduction (abducted 90° and elbow flexed 90°) (70°).

Power

- Abduction against resistance (deltoid): axillary nerve palsy ⇒ loss of deltoid activity and loss of sensation in 'regimental badge' area;
- Push against wall (serratus anterior): long thoracic nerve palsy ⇒ winged scapula.

Special tests
Rotator cuff:

= supraspinatus and infraspinatus and subscapularis and teres minor. Assess for *pain* (rotator cuff tendinitis) and *weakness* (rotator cuff tear)

- *Supraspinatus test*: resisted abduction with arm in maximal internal rotation + 20° abduction + 20° flexion (supraspinatus tear: cannot initiate abduction and ↓ external rotation).
- *Infraspinatus test*
  - resisted external rotation with elbow flexed to 90°;
  - good general test of rotator test function.
- *Subscapularis tests*
  - resisted internal rotation with elbow flexed to 90°;
  - lift-off test (Gerber's test): shoulder internally rotated with arm behind back and hand resisted from lifting off posteriorly.
- *Drop arm test*
  - shoulder abducted 90°;
  - patient lowers arm gradually with examiner applying gentle pressure;
  - unable to control lowering (arm drops) at ~30° ⇒ rotator cuff tear.

- *Biceps tests*
    - resisted elbow flexion with forearm in neutral rotation (biceps bulges if long head ruptured);
    - resisted forward flexion of shoulder with elbow extended and forearm supinated (Speed's test);
    - resisted supination with elbow flexed to 90° (Yergason's test).

ACJ (localization of pain).
- *ACJ stress test*
    - forced passive adduction across chest with arm flexed to 90°;
    - injection of 1% lignocaine into ACJ relieves pain.

Impingement

- *Painful arc*: pain in arc of 60–120° of abduction ⇒ impingement;
- *Impingement sign* (Neer)
    - forced passive forward flexion (acromion fixed);
    - pain at 90° abduction ⇒ impingement.
- *Impingement test* (Neer)
    - 5–10 ml 1% lignocaine injected into subacromial space;
    - repeat above manoeuvre after 10 min;
    - assess for abolition of pain.
- *Hawkins' test*: forward flexion to 90° and forced internal rotation.
- *Jobe's test*: forward flexion to 30° and abduction to 90° against resistance.

Instability

Observe any translation of joint or degree of patient apprehension.
- *Anterior apprehension test*
    - patient sits or lies supine with shoulder abducted 90°;
    - grasp elbow with one hand and place other hand over shoulder;
    - apply gradual external rotation in extension;
    - thumb gently pushes humeral head forward;
    - look for apprehension/feel for pectoral muscle spasm;
    - suggests anterior instability or impingement;
    - can repeat with shoulder in various degrees of abduction.
- *Relocation test (Jobe)*
    - push proximal humerus backwards and repeat apprehension manoeuvre;
    - no apprehension ⇒ instability (application of an anterior stabilizing force allows further external rotation);
    - continuing apprehension ⇒ impingement.

- *Inferior subluxation test*
    - patient sits with arms hanging relaxed;
    - apply downward traction on arm;
    - look for sulcus between acromion and humeral head (sulcus sign).
- *Posterior stress test*
    - patient sits with shoulder adducted and internally rotated.
    - palpate glenohumeral joint posteriorly.
    - push humeral head posteriorly by holding elbow and applying axial loading to the humerus.
    - forward flex arm 90° (feel for posterior subluxation)
    - then continue manoeuvre by abducting the 90° flexed shoulder (clunk $\Rightarrow$ reduction of posterior subluxation).
- *Anterior/posterior drawer test*
    - patient sits with forearm resting in lap;
    - stabilize scapula with one hand;
    - firmly grip humeral head with other hand;
    - attempt to translate humeral head forwards and backwards;
    - can repeat with shoulder in various degrees of abduction.

X-ray

AP (in plane of shoulder - 30° anterior to the coronal plane).
- Axillary lateral (arm abducted 70-90°) *or* scapular lateral.

Additional views
- Hill-Sachs lesion (posterolateral defect of humeral head suggestive of anterior instability)
    - AP in >50° internal rotation;
    - Stryker notch view: AP with tube tilted 10° upwards and patient's hand on head;
    - West Point view: axillary lateral with patient prone and tube tilted 25° downwards and 25° medially.
- ACJ: AP with tube tilted 20° upwards ± patient holding a weight on the affected side (may need comparison view of uninjured side).

Alternative imaging
- MRI.
- CT/CT arthrogram.

Assessment of shoulder radiographs

- *Adequacy*: good lateral required to exclude posterior glenohumeral dislocation.
- *Alignment*
    - glenohumeral joint
        - congruent joint surfaces (AP or axillary lateral);
        - humeral head centred over 'Mercedes star' (scapular lateral).
    - ACJ.

- *Bones*
    - humerus (head, neck);
    - scapula (glenoid, acromion, coracoid, blade);
    - clavicle.
- Cartilage and joints (joint space).
- Soft tissues: calcification in supraspinatus tendon.

EXAMINATION OF THE ELBOW

- Introduce yourself to the patient.
- Ask the patient for permission to perform an examination.
- Adequately expose both elbows, wrists and hands.
- Ask patient if their elbow is painful.

Look

(a) Arms held straight alongside body with palms facing forwards.

(b) Arms held with shoulders abducted 90° and elbows extended and palms facing upwards.

- Skin: scars, colour changes.
- Shape
    - swelling: olecranon bursa, joint (loss of concavities on either side of olecranon);
    - wasting;
    - deformity (abnormal carrying angle, fixed flexion);
        - carrying angle = valgus angle between arm and forearm with elbow full extended;
        - normal average = 11° (males), 13° (females);
        - altered by fracture malunion or epiphyseal injury;
        - cubitus valgus = ↑ carrying angle, ulnar nerve palsy common;
        - cubitus varus ('gun-stock' deformity) = ↓ carrying angle.
- Position: resting position.

- Compare with the opposite elbow.

Feel

- Skin: temperature.
- Soft tissues
    - lumps, thickening, wasting;
    - crepitus ⇒ tenosynovitis);
    - nodules (rheumatoid).
- Bones and joints
    - outlines (olecranon and both epicondyles form a nearly equilateral triangle in 90° flexion and straight line in extension);

- synovial thickening;
- loose bodies;
- fluid swelling (fluctuation on either side of olecranon).
- Tenderness
    - lateral epicondyle ('tennis elbow');
    - medial epicondyle ('golfer's' elbow);
    - olecranon;
    - radial head;
    - anterior elbow joint (either side of biceps tendon);
    - ulnar nerve behind medial epicondyle.

Move
Normal range of movement (see Diagram 13).

Passive/active
- Flexion (140°).
- Extension (0°)/hyperextension (up to -15° in young females).
- Pronation (elbow flexed 90° and held at side) (75°).
- Supination (elbow flexed 90° and held at side) (80°).

Special tests
- Tennis elbow
    - extend elbow with hand fully pronated;
    - pronate hand with elbow fully extended;
    - resisted dorsiflexion of clenched fist with elbow fully extended.
- Golfer's elbow: extend elbow with hand fully supinated.
- Ulnar nerve
    - tenderness/palpable thickening of nerve behind medial epicondyle;
    - reproduction of paraesthesia on tapping over nerve (Tinel's sign).
- Instability
    - varus/valgus
        - flex elbow 20-30°;
        - apply varus stress with arm internally rotated;
        - apply valgus stress with arm externally rotated.

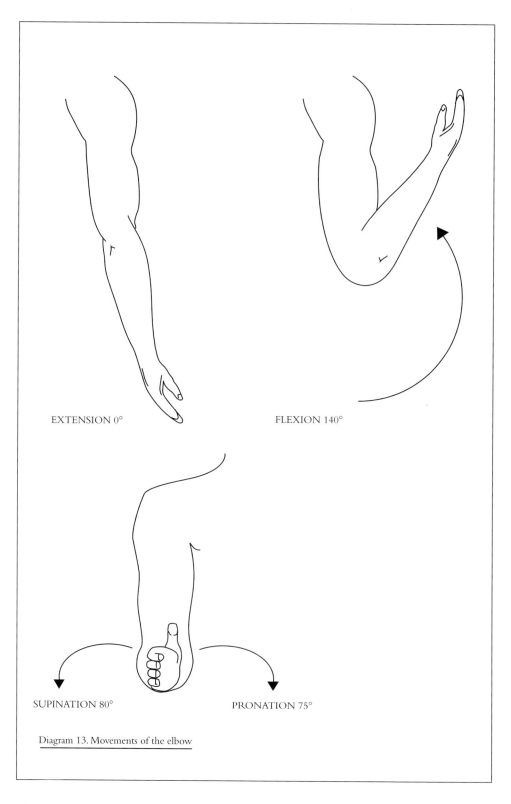

EXTENSION 0°

FLEXION 140°

SUPINATION 80°

PRONATION 75°

Diagram 13. Movements of the elbow

- lateral pivot shift test
  - start with elbow flexed 90°;
  - fully supinate forearm;
  - apply valgus and supination and axial compression forces;
  - slowly extend elbow;
  - posterolateral subluxation of radiohumeral joint $\Rightarrow$ posterolateralrotatory instability.

X-ray
- AP (elbow extended).
- Lateral (elbow flexed to 90°).

Additional views
- Obliques (radial head and distal humerus fractures).
- AP in supination and pronation (radial head fractures).

Assessment of elbow radiographs
- Adequacy.
- Alignment
  - anterior humeral and central radial lines intersect middle of capitellum (lateral view).
  - elbow joint: congruent joint surfaces.
- Bones
  - humerus;
  - radius;
  - ulna.
- Cartilage and joints (joint space).
- Soft tissues: anterior and posterior fat pads (fat displaced by an effusion $\Rightarrow$ triangular-shaped radiolucent shadow adjacent to distal humerus on lateral view).

Secondary ossification centres around the elbow
(appearance $\rightarrow$ fusion, in years of age).
- Capitellum: 2 $\rightarrow$ 18.
- Radial head: 4 $\rightarrow$ 18.
- Medial epicondyle: 5 $\rightarrow$ 18.
- Trochlea: 9 $\rightarrow$ 18.
- Olecranon: 10 $\rightarrow$ 18.
- Lateral epicondyle: 12 $\rightarrow$ 18.

EXAMINATION OF THE WRIST

Anatomy

Carpal bones: two rows (from radial to ulnar)
- Proximal: scaphoid, lunate, triquetrum, pisiform.
- Distal: trapezoid, capitate, hamate.

Joints
- Radiocarpal joint – between distal radius and scaphoid/lunate/triquetrum.
- Ulnocarpal joint – primarily composed of the triangular fibrocartilage complex (TFCC).
- Distal radioulnar joint (DRUJ).
- Intercarpal joints.

- Introduce yourself to the patient.
- Ask the patient for permission to perform an examination.
- Ask the patient to show both wrists and hands.
- Ask the patient if their wrist is painful.

Look
- Skin: scars, colour changes.
- Shape: swelling (subcutaneous tissue, tendon sheath, joint), wasting, deformity.
- Position: resting position.

- Compare with the opposite wrist (record pattern of joint involvement, if polyarticular).

Feel
Note any tenderness.
- (Skin: temperature, moisture).
- Soft tissues
    - lumps, thickening, wasting;
    - crepitus ($\Rightarrow$ tenosynovitis);
    - nodules (rheumatoid, stenosing tenovaginitis).
- Bones and joints: outlines, synovium, fluid swelling (fluctuance on dorsum of wrist).

Move

Normal range of movement (*see **Diagram 14***).

Passive ± active:
- Dorsiflexion (70°). Comparison: place both palms together in position of prayer and raise elbows.
- Palmarflexion (75°). Comparison: place dorsum of both hands together and lower elbows.
- Radial deviation (20°).
- Ulnar deviation (35°).
- Pronation (elbow flexed 90° and held at side) (75°).
- Supination (elbow flexed 90° and held at side) (80°).

Special tests
- Piano key test
    - stabilize distal radius and move head of ulna in AP direction;
    - mobility/pain/crepitus ⇒ distal radioulnar joint instability.
- Scaphoid shift (Kirk Watson's test)
    - push on palmar aspect of distal pole of scaphoid;
      wrist: dorsiflexion and ulnar deviation ⇒ palmar flexion and radial deviation;
    - pain/clunk ⇒ scapholunate instability.
- Finkelstein's test
    - passive ulnar deviation of wrist with fingers closed over flexed thumb;
    - pain ⇒ de Quervain's disease (stenosing tenovaginitis of extensor pollicis brevis/abductor pollicis longus) or degenerative arthritis of 1st CMCJ (trapezio-metacarpal joint).
- Grind test
    - hold thumb MCPJ;
    - forcefully push and rotate thumb metacarpal against 1st CMCJ;
    - pain ⇒ degenerative arthritis of 1st CMCJ.
- Tinel's sign
    - reproduction of paraesthesia on tapping over nerve;
    - e.g. tapping over median nerve at wrist in carpal tunnel syndrome.
- Phalen's sign
    - full palmarflexion of wrist held for 1 min;
    - reproduction of paraesthesia ⇒ carpal tunnel syndrome.

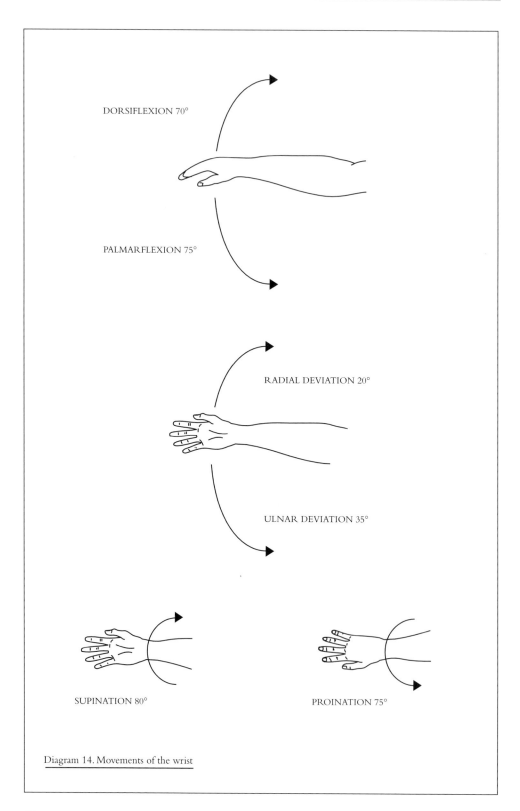

DORSIFLEXION 70°

PALMARFLEXION 75°

RADIAL DEVIATION 20°

ULNAR DEVIATION 35°

SUPINATION 80°

PROINATION 75°

Diagram 14. Movements of the wrist

X-ray

- PA.
- Lateral.

Additional views
- Scaphoid views
    - PA in ulnar deviation;
    - Lateral in neutral;
    - Semipronated (PA) oblique in ulnar deviation;
    - Semisupinated (AP) oblique in ulnar deviation.
- Stress views
    - PA in radial deviation;
    - PA in ulnar deviation;
    - PA supinated with clenched fist;
    - lateral with clenched fist.
- Tangential views (foreign bodies).

Assessment of wrist radiographs

- Adequacy
    - PA: no overlap between distal radius and ulna;
    - lateral: distal radius and ulna superimposed.
- Alignment
    - PA
        - proximal and distal carpal rows;
        - articular surfaces of distal radius and distal radius should form a smooth line.
    - lateral:
        - 10-15° volar tilt of radiocarpal joint.
        - A line should bisect distal radius, lunate, capitate, middle metacarpal base (wrist in neutral position).
- Bones
    - distal carpal row;
    - proximal carpal row;
    - distal radius and ulna.
- Cartilage and joints (joint space).
    - radiocarpal joint;
    - distal radioulnar joint;
    - scapholunate interval (PA supinated clenched fist view): >3 mm (Terry-Thomas sign) ⇒ scapholunate dissociation.

- scapholunate angle (lateral view):
  - $>60°$ $\Rightarrow$ DISI (dorsal intercalated segment instability).
  - $<30°$ $\Rightarrow$ VISI (volar intercalated segment instability).
- Soft tissues.

EXAMINATION OF THE HAND

Anatomy
- Hand and each digit
    - dorsal and volar (or palmar) surfaces;
    - radial and ulnar borders.
- Palm
    - thenar eminence;
    - mid-palm;
    - hypothenar eminence.
- Each finger
    - metacarpophalangeal joint (MCPJ);
    - proximal interphalangeal joint (PIPJ);
    - distal interphalangeal joint (DIPJ).
- Thumb
    - metacarpophalangeal joint (MCPJ);
    - interphalangeal joint (IPJ).

The thumb's carpometacarpal joint (CMCJ) is unique in its mobility.

Two main hand functions
- *Pinch grip*: opposition of thumb and any other finger (usually index finger).
- *Power grip*: mainly involves ulnar three fingers flexing against palm of hand.

- Introduce yourself to the patient.
- Ask the patient for permission to perform an examination.
- Ask the patient to show both hands.
- Ask the patient if their hand is painful.

Look
- Skin: scars, colour changes.
- Shape: swelling (subcutaneous tissue, tendon sheath, joint), muscle wasting, deformity.
- Position: resting position. Extended finger in suspected tendon injury ⇒ division of FDS and FDP.
- Compare with the opposite limb (record pattern of joint involvement if polyarticular).

Feel

Note any tenderness.

- Skin
    - temperature, moisture;
    - sensation (light touch, pinprick, two-point discrimination);
        - ulnar nerve: little finger;
        - median nerve: index finger;
        - radial nerve: lateral aspect of base of thumb.
- Soft tissues
    - lumps, thickening, wasting;
    - crepitus ($\Rightarrow$ tenosynovitis);
    - nodules in palm (rheumatoid, stenosing tenovaginitis).
- Bones and joints: outlines, synovium, fluid swelling.

- Vascularity
    - radial and ulnar pulses;
    - capillary refill of nail bed;
    - Allen's test (see below).

Move

- Active
    - Full flexion (make fist with palm upwards - check for full 'tuck-in'): flexion deficit = distance from fingertip to palm.
    - Full extension (palm downward).
    - Grip strength
        - squeeze examiner's hand;
        - squeeze sphygmomanometer cuff inflated to 50 mmHg (normal $\uparrow$ to >150 mmHg).
    - Nerve function (active movements against resistance)
        - ulnar nerve: finger abduction, thumb adduction (Froment's sign – see below);
        - median nerve: thumb abduction;
        - radial nerve: finger and thumb MCPJ extension.
    - Tendon function (active movements against resistance)
        - FDS tendon: PIPJ flexion (hold other fingers extended);
        - FDP tendon: DIPJ flexion (hold PIPJ extended);
        - extensor tendons: finger and thumb MCPJ extension (already tested).
- Passive (normal range of movement) **(see Diagram 15).**

FINGER FLEXION

MCPJ 85°(Index)
105°(Middle)

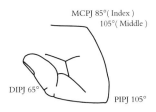

DIPJ 65°

PIPJ 105°

FINGER EXTENSION

DIPJ 0°

PIPJ 0°

MCPJ 20°

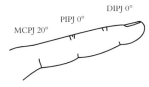

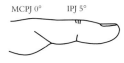

THUMB EXTENSION

MCPJ 0°   IPJ 5°

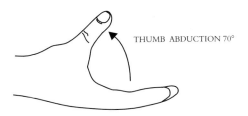

THUMB FLEXION

MCPJ 50°

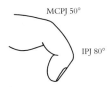

IPJ 80°

THUMB ABDUCTION 70°

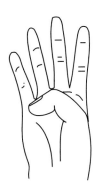

THUMB OPPOSITION
thumb tip reaches base of the little finger

Diagram 15. Movements of the hand

- Range of movement of each digit
  - finger flexion (MCPJ 85° for index to 105° for little), PIPJ 105°;
  - DIPJ 65° ;
  - finger extension (MCPJ 20°, PIPJ 0°, DIPJ 0°);
  - thumb flexion (MCPJ 60°, IPJ 80°);
  - thumb extension (MCPJ 0°, IPJ 5°);
  - thumb abduction (70°);
  - thumb opposition (base of little finger).
- Intrinsic tightness: compare PIPJ flexion with MCPJs flexed and extended. ↓ PIPJ flexion with MCPJs extended ⇒ intrinsic tightness (e.g. post-traumatic contracture).
- Abnormal movements (instability): fingers show side-to-side stability in 90° flexion (collateral ligaments tightened).

Special tests
- Allen's test
  - patient elevates hand and makes a fist;
  - compress radial and ulnar arteries at wrist;
  - patient exsanguinates hand by opening and closing fist several times;
  - release radial artery;
  - 'pinking' of hand in <5 s ⇒ patency of radial artery;
  - repeat with release of ulnar artery.
- Froment's sign
  - patient asked to hold piece of paper between thumb and index finger;
  - thumb IPJ flexion rather than thumb adduction used ⇒ ulnar nerve palsy.

Flexor tendon injuries
Site of flexor tendon injury may be in one of five zones.
Zone 2 (distal palmar crease → PIPJ) is most important
- FDS and FDP tendons are injured in their sheath;
- high risk of poor healing with adhesions between the two tendons and sheath.

The rheumatoid hand
- Stage 1
  - symmetrical tender swelling of MCPJs, IPJs and wrist;
  - swelling of tendon sheaths (ext. carpi ulnaris, flexor tendons);
  - ↓ joint mobility;

- ↓ grip strength;
- carpal tunnel compression.
- Stage 2: early deformities
  - radial tilt and volar subluxation of wrist;
  - ulnar deviation of fingers;
  - swan-neck deformity (PIPJ hyperextension and DIPJ flexion);
  - boutonniére deformity (PIPJ flexion and DIPJ hyperextension);
  - drop finger/mallet thumb (extensor tendon rupture);
  - Z deformity of thumb (MCPJ flexion and IPJ hyperextension).
- Stage 3: established deformities (as above) → dislocations and loss of function.

X-ray
- PA.
- Oblique.
- True lateral.

Additional views
- PA and lateral views of single digit (if injury/disease confined to distal end of a digit).
- PA and lateral views of thumb.
- Tangential views (foreign bodies).

Assessment of hand radiographs
- Adequacy.
- Alignment: follow alignment of phalanges and metacarpal for each digit.
- Bones
  - thumb;
  - fingers;
  - metacarpals;
  - wrist.
- Cartilage and joints (joint space).
- Soft tissues.

EXAMINATION OF THE HIP

2-

- Introduce yourself to the patient.
- Ask the patient for permission to perform an examination.
- Adequately expose both lower limbs.
- Do not expose external genitalia (consider a patient's privacy in the examination setting).
- Ask the patient if their hip is painful.

Patient standing
Look
- Gait (observe patient walking from in front and behind)
    - antalgic: $\downarrow$ stance phase and $\uparrow$ swing phase.
    - short leg: ipsilateral hip sinks when weight is on short leg.
    - Trendelenburg
        - ipsilateral hip dips when leg raised;
        - usually associated with compensatory lurch of trunk;
        - due to poor contralateral abductor function.
    - neuropathic: e.g. broad-based gait (cerebellar ataxia), scissoring gait (spasticity).
- Trendelenburg test
    - patient stands on one leg (normal side first) with other leg flexed at knee;
    - repeat with patient standing on abnormal leg;
    - +ve on supported side if hip dips on unsupported side $\Rightarrow$ weak abductors, dislocated hip, shortened neck of femur, painful hip;
    - Trendelenburg lurch: body thrown over affected hip to compensate.
- Posture: pelvic tilt, $\uparrow$ lumbar lordosis.

Patient supine
Look
- Skin: scars, sinuses, skin creases.
- Shape: swelling, muscle wasting (quadriceps, gluteal muscles).
- Position
    - apparent leg lengths (tape measurement: xiphisternum $\Rightarrow$ medial malleolus);

- fixed deformity
  - fixed adduction deformity → apparent leg shortening;
  - fixed abduction deformity → apparent leg lengthening.

Measure

- Limb length
  - check pelvis is square (with patient lying along midline of couch, thumbs under ASISs should lie on imaginary transverse line a cross couch);
  - if unable to square up pelvis: 'correct' deformity by placing normal leg in same position as abnormal leg;
  - assess true limb length;
  - difference between levels of medial malleoli (rough measurement only);
  - tape measurement: ASIS → medial malleolus.
- Locate any discrepancy
  - above/below knee: Galeazzi test - flex knees so that feet lie flat on bed with heels perfectly together and look from the side (± measure medial malleolus → medial joint line of knee);
  - above/below greater trochanter (*see Diagram 16*);
  - bilateral palpation (thumbs under ASISs, middle fingers on GTs);
  - Nélaton's line (passes through top of GT with hip flexed and adducted);
  - Bryant's triangle (compare x on each side).

Feel

- (Skin: temperature.)
- (Soft tissues: contours.)
- Bones and joints: feel for resistance of femoral head in groin.
- Tenderness
  - femoral head (deep palpation over midpoint of inguinal ligament);
  - adductor longus insertion;
  - lesser trochanter;
  - greater trochanter (and trochanteric bursa);
  - ischial tuberosity.
- Peripheral pulses: dorsalis pedis and posterior tibial.

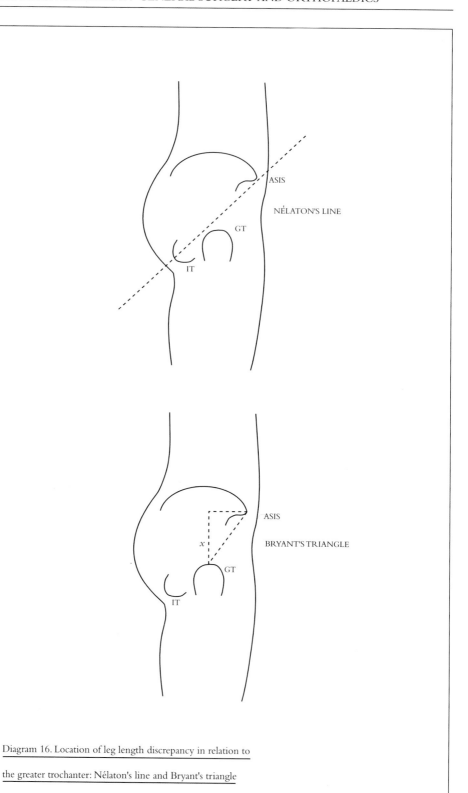

Diagram 16. Location of leg length discrepancy in relation to

the greater trochanter: Nélaton's line and Bryant's triangle

Move

- Normal range of movement (*see Diagram 17*).
- Movements usually only tested passively.
- Lumbar lordosis and tilting of pelvis may cause inaccuracy.

- Flexion (120°)
- Thomas' test
- Tests for fixed flexion deformity;
    - flex both hips to comfortable position;
    - maximally flex normal hip;
    - feel for flattening of lumbar lordosis;
    - maintain maximum flexion of normal hip (can ask patient to hold onto knee);
    - allow abnormal hip to drop into extension;
    - look for fixed flexion of abnormal hip.
- (Extension (10°): with patient prone or on side.)
- Abduction (40°)
    - place hand on opposite ASIS to detect tilting of pelvis;
    - can fix pelvis by abducting 'good' hip over edge of table;
    - in children: test abduction in flexion.
- Adduction (30°)
    - move leg over opposite leg or lift up opposite leg;
    - measure with respect to opposite patella.
- Internal/external rotation (40°/40°)
    - (a) in extension with knees extended: compare movement of patellae;
    - (b) in 90° hip flexion with knees flexed 90°.

- Abnormal movement ('telescoping')
    - stabilize pelvis with one hand;
    - pull up on 90° flexed hip using other hand behind flexed knee.

Special tests

- DDH (developmental dysplasia of the hip; also known as CDH = congenital dislocation of the hip)
    - Ortolani's test (dislocated hip)
        - both knees grasped with hips and knees flexed;
        - +ve: clunk of relocation on abduction of 90° flexed hip.
    - Barlow's test (dislocatable hip)
        - one hand holds pelvis with thumb on pubic symphysis and fingers on sacrum;
        - other hand holds one leg with knee flexed 90° and tip of middle finger on GT;

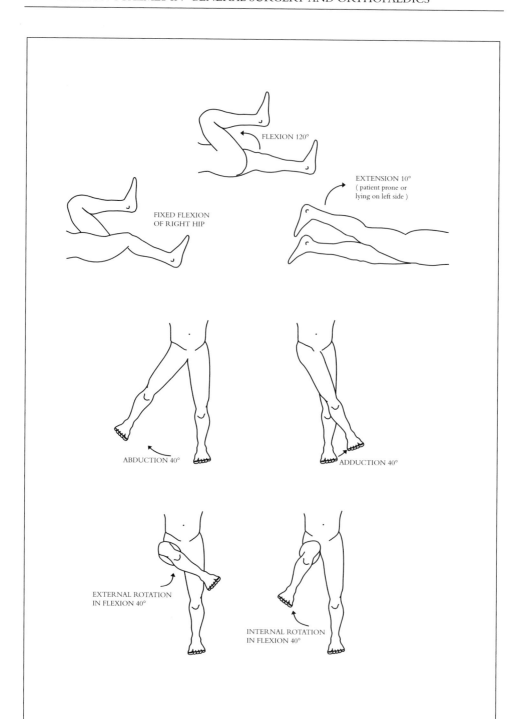

Diagram 17. Movements of the hip

- +ve: subluxation with firm backward pressure on flexed and adducted hip;
- subsequent abduction ⇒ reduction clunk.

- Gauvain's test
  - forced internal rotation of hip;
  - reflex abdominal muscle contraction ⇒ painful hip condition.

Patient Prone
- Look: skin, shape, position.
- Feel: muscle wasting.
- Move
  - extension (10°)
    - active (check quality of glutei);
    - passive.
  - internal/external rotation with knees flexed 90° (40°/40°).

Rotational profile (children)
- Foot progression angle (FPA): angle of foot during gait (normal 0-5° external rotation).
- Foot-thigh angle (FTA)
  - flex knee 90° with patient prone and look down from above;
  - tibial torsion (internal or external) = angle between longitudinal axis of foot and longitudinal axis of thigh;
  - (normal slight internal tibial torsion in infancy → external tibial torsion of 10-15° at maturity.)
- Range of hip rotation
  - patient prone with knees flexed 90°;
  - rotate hip internally and externally (normal internal/external rotation: infancy 70°/35° → maturity 40°/40°);
  - femoral anteversion = angle of internal rotation of hip when GT is most prominent.

X-ray
- AP pelvis.
- Lateral hip (cross-table).

Additional views
- AP with 15° internal rotation (femoral neck).
- Frog lateral (children).

- Oblique (undisplaced femoral neck fractures, trochanteric fractures).
- CDH: AP with full internal rotation and >45° abduction.
- Pelvic fracture: inlet and outlet views (AP with tube tilted 30-45° caudad and cephalad respectively).
- Acetabular fracture: Judet views (45° internal [obturator] oblique to show anterior column/posterior acetabulum and 45° external [iliac] oblique to show posterior column/anterior acetabulum).

Assessment of AP pelvis radiograph

- Adequacy
  - whole pelvis included: iliac crests, both hips, femurs distal to lesser trochanters;
  - rotation (pubic symphysis lined up over midline of sacrum);
  - both hips should be symmetrical.
- Alignment
  - trace around three rings pelvic brim +both obturator foramina
    - look for fracture or diastasis;
    - pelvic ring must disrupt in more than one place;
    - pubic symphysis widening >2.5 cm $\Rightarrow$ SIJ involved.
  - Shenton's line (smooth arc formed by superior border of obturator foramen and inferior border of femoral neck);
  - medial $\frac{1}{2}$ of femoral head overlaps posterior acetabular rim.
- Bones
  - superior and inferior pubic rami;
  - ilium (including iliac crest);
  - sacrum (trace around sacral foramina);
  - lumbar vertebrae;
  - femoral head and rest of proximal femur (especially neck and trochanters).
- Cartilage and joints (joint space)
  - pubic symphysis (widening, overlapping);
  - sacroiliac joints (widening, cortical defects, overlapping, incongruity);
  - acetabulum
    - posterior joint margin;
    - anterior joint margin;
    - posterior column (ilioischial line);
    - anterior column (iliopectineal line);
    - tear drop (acetabular floor).
- Soft tissues: inside and outside pelvis.

EXAMINATION OF THE KNEE

- Introduce yourself to the patient.
- Ask the patient for permission to perform an examination.
- Adequately expose both lower limbs.
- Ask the patient if their knee is painful.

Patient standing
Look.

Gait (observe patient walking from in front and behind)
- antalgic: ↓ stance phase;
- stiff knee gait: pelvis rises to provide clearance during swing phase;
- instability (thrust) gait: may be mechanical or neuropathic.
- Alignment
  - neutral;
  - varus/valgus (can measure intermalleolar or interknee distance);
  - fixed flexion;
  - hyperextension (recurvatum).
- Popliteal fossa

Special test
- Meniscal tear
  - squat test: patient performs full squats with legs internally and externally rotated
    - medial pain/pain in external rotation ⇒ medial meniscal tear;
    - lateral pain/pain in internal rotation ⇒ lateral meniscal tear.

Patient supine
Look

- Skin: discoloration, sinuses, scars.
- Shape
  - alignment (see above);
  - quadriceps wasting (especially vastus medialis);
  - joint effusion (compare hollows on either side and above patella);
  - bony swelling;
  - patellar alignment (neutral, subluxed, dislocated, absent);
  - Q-angle (valgus angle formed by ASIS and midpoint of patella and tibial

tuberosity) measured with knee fully extended: 15° in females, 10° in males – ↑ angle predisposes to patellar instability.
- Position: check for fixed flexion.

Feel
- Skin: temperature (palm of hand: proximal thigh to distal leg).
- Effusion (empty suprapatellar pouch first by expressing fluid distally using 1st web space)
    - sweep (stroke) test: anchor patella, empty medial side by sweeping back of hand up medial side of knee, then sweep hand down lateral side;
    - patellar tap: push patella posteriorly against femoral condyles;
    - cross-fluctuation: squeeze each side alternately.
- Soft tissues
    - quadriceps wasting
        - palpate contracted muscle bulk (especially vastus medialis) with patient pushing knee back into couch;
        - measure thigh circumference a set distance (e.g. 15 cm) above joint line and compare with opposite side.
    - quadriceps tendon.
    - patellar tendon.
    - synovial thickening (especially proximal edge of suprapatellar pouch).
- Bones and joints
    - patellar alignment;
    - joint line (knee flexed to 90°, foot flat on couch).
- Tenderness
    - joint line;
    - collateral ligaments;
    - tibial tuberosity;
    - femoral condyles;
    - margins of patella;
    - retropatellar;
    - popliteal fossa (patient prone): Baker's cyst, popliteal artery aneurysm.
- Peripheral pulses: dorsalis pedis and posterior tibial.

Move
Normal range of movement (*see Diagram 18*)

Active

- flexion;
- extension;
- (rotation);
- straight leg raise (tests integrity of extensor mechanism): look for extensor lag and fixed flexion deformity.

Passive

- flexion (140° - normally limited by apposition of hamstring and calf muscles)
    - place hand over patella and note any crepitus, clicks;
- extension (0°)/hyperextension (up to - 10° of recurvatum)
    - record range of movement as: hyperextension/full extension (0°)/flexion, e.g. 10° of fixed flexion deformity is 0°/10°/140°;
    - distinguish fixed flexion from springy block to extension (occurs in any painful knee condition).
- (rotation)
    - can measure heel-buttock distance.

Abnormal movements (ensure patient is relaxed)
Standard stress tests

Collateral ligaments
- *Varus/valgus stress*
    - with knee flexed 20-30°, apply alternate varus and valgus stress with one hand at knee and one hand holding the ankle; *or* with knee flexed 20-30° and index fingers on femoral condyles, apply stress via patient's lower leg in examiner's axilla;
    - repeat varus and valgus stress with knee in full extension. Instability in extension ⇒ cruciate and collateral ligament disruption.

Cruciate ligaments (ensure quadriceps and hamstrings are relaxed)
- *Posterior sag*
    - flex knees 70-90°, keeping feet flat on couch *or* flex hips and knees 90° and support heels in examiner's hands;
    - look across anterior profile of both knees.
    'Drop back' or sag ⇒ PCL rupture.

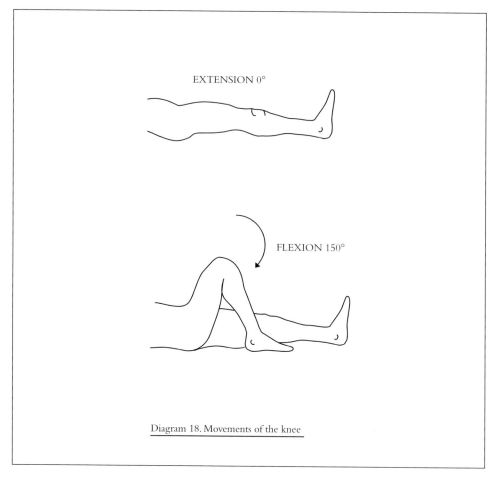

EXTENSION 0°

FLEXION 150°

Diagram 18. Movements of the knee

- *Anterior/posterior drawer* (tests anteroposterior instability)
  - flex knee 70-90° and sit on foot to stabilize it;
  - place hands behind knee (feel for hamstring relaxation);
  - pull tibia forwards (anterior drawer) and push tibia backwards (posterior drawer)
    - 1+ = 0-5 mm, 2+ = 6-10 mm;
    - 3+ = 11-15 mm, 4+ >15 mm;
    - end-point: firm ($\Rightarrow$ ACL intact), marginal, soft posterior sag $\Rightarrow$ false +ve anterior drawer test (but –ve pivot shift test).
- *Lachman test* (useful test of ACL integrity if knee painful or swollen)
  - with knee flexed 20° hold distal thigh firmly with one hand and lift proximal tibia forward with other hand (thumb on anteromedial joint line): *or* flex knee over examiner's thigh, press down on distal

thigh and lift proximal tibia forward
  - 1+ = 0-5 mm, 2+ = 6-10 mm;
  - 3+ = 11-15 mm, 4+ >15 mm;
  - end-point: firm ($\Rightarrow$ ACL intact), marginal, soft.
- Meniscal tear
  - *McMurray's test*
    - flex knee maximally, grasp knee with one hand and foot with other;
    - medial meniscus: palpate posteromedial joint line and externally rotate leg;
    - lateral meniscus: palpate posterolateral joint line and internally rotate leg;
    - slowly extend knee;
    - palpable click $\Rightarrow$ meniscal tear
      at full flexion to 90° $\Rightarrow$ posterior peripheral tear;
    - at 90° to full extension $\Rightarrow$ middle or anterior tear;
    - pain during the test is also suggestive of a meniscal tear;
    - repeat with varus and valgus stress applied.

Special tests
- Rotary tests of cruciate ligaments
  - *Pivot shift test* (MacIntosh): test of anterolateral instability
    - with knee extended and tibia internally rotated by examiner's hand holding ankle, exert valgus strain with hand over proximal fibula, then slowly flex knee 20-30° (to reduce anteriorly sub-luxed tibia).
      No movement, grind, 1+ (glide), 2+ (clunk), 3+ (gross);
    - can also add axial compressive force to knee either using hand holding ankle or pushing patient's foot against examiner's thigh.
  - *Reverse pivot shift*: test of posterolateral instability: as pivot shift test but tibia externally rotated and extend knee from 30° flexion (to reduce posteriorly subluxed tibia);
  - *Anterior rotary drawer test* (Slocum)
    - repeat anterior drawer test
      - in 15° internal rotation (posterolateral capsule tightened: test of anterolateral instability);
      - in 30° external rotation (posteromedial capsule tightened: test of anteromedial instability).

- *Jerk test* (Hughston and Losee)
  - with knee flexed 90° and tibia internally rotated, apply valgus strain with hand over proximal fibula and gradually extend knee;
  - +ve: lateral tibia spontaneously subluxes forward (as a jerk) at ~30° flexion.
- Patellar instability
  - *Patella tracking*
    - observe mobility of patella as patient slowly extends knee. +ve J sign: slight lateral subluxation of patella as knee approaches full extension;
    - with knee extended and relaxed, patient tightens quadriceps. Normal: patella moves more superiorly than laterally.
  - *Patellar apprehension test*
    - with knee extended, push patella laterally and slowly flex knee 10-20°,
    - quadriceps contraction ⇒ recurrent patellar subluxation.
  - *Patellar tilt test*
    - flex knee 20°;
    - use thumb to flip lateral edge of patella away from femoral condyle;
    - little upward movement ⇒ tight lateral retinaculum.
  - *Patellar friction test* (chondromalacia patellae)
    - knee rests extended;
    - press patella backwards and distally onto patellofemoral groove;
    - patient then gently contracts quadriceps;
    - pain ⇒ chondromalacia patellae (Clarke's sign).
- *Larson test* (osteochondritis dissecans)
  - with knee flexed and internally rotated, gradually extend knee;
  - pain ⇒ osteochondritis dissecans of medial femoral condyle.
- *Popliteal angle* (measure of hamstring tightness): angle of tibia from vertical with patient supine, hip flexed 90° and knee extended maximally.

Patient prone
- **Look**: popliteal fossa.
- **Feel**: popliteal fossa (with knee slightly flexed to reduce soft tissue tension).

Special test
- Meniscal tear
  - Apley grinding test

- patient lies prone;
- with knee flexed 90°, fix thigh against couch;
- pull leg upwards by foot and rotate, pain $\Rightarrow$ ligament injury;
- press leg downwards by foot and rotate as knee is flexed and extended, pain $\Rightarrow$ meniscal tear.

X-ray
- AP: preferably weight-bearing.
- Lateral: horizontal beam required in trauma patients to detect lipohaemarthrosis (fat-blood fluid level in suprapatellar pouch).

Additional views
- Tangential patellar views (assessment of patellofemoral joint).
    - skyline: tangential beam with knee flexed 30°;
    - Merchant view: axial view with knee flexed 45°, X-ray beam at 30° to horizontal and cassette held perpendicular to tibia.
- Tunnel (intercondylar notch): PA view with knee partly flexed.
- AP views with varus and valgus stress.
- Frontal oblique views in internal and external rotation (to assess tibial plateaux).
- Arthrogram.

Assessment of knee radiographs
- Adequacy
- Alignment
    - congruent articulation between femoral condyles and tibial plateau;
    - femoral/tibial angle;
    - patella: lies anterior to proximal portion of femoral condyles (lateral view). There are three methods of assessing patella alta (high-riding patella) or patella baja (low-riding patella)
        - Insall-Salvati index: ratio of patellar tendon length to patella length; >1.2 = patella alta, <0.8 = patella baja/infera;
        - Blackburne and Peel index: ratio of (a) distance from tibial plateau to inferior articular surface of patella, to (b) length of patella articular surface; normal = 0.8, >1.0 = patella alta;
        - Blumensaat line: line extended from intercondylar notch with knee flexed 30°; normal: lower pole of patella lies on intercondylar line.

- Bones
    - distal femur;
    - proximal tibia;
    - patella;
    - proximal fibula.
- Cartilage and joints (joint space, loose bodies)
    - medial compartment;
    - lateral compartment;
    - patellofemoral joint.
- Soft tissues
    - effusion;
    - lipohaemarthrosis;
    - chondrocalcinosis (meniscal calcification $\Rightarrow$ OA, pseudogout);
    - surgical emphysema;
    - foreign bodies.

Other investigations
- Aspiration
    - blood $\Rightarrow$ ACL tear;
    - blood and fat globules $\Rightarrow$ intra-articular fracture.
- MRI.
- Diagnostic arthroscopy.

EXAMINATION OF THE ANKLE AND FOOT

Anatomy
- Hindfoot: calcaneum and talus.
- Midfoot: navicular and cuboid and cuneiforms.
- Forefoot: metatarsals and phalanges.

- Subtalar joint = anterior talocalcaneal joint and talonavicular joint.
- Mid-tarsal joint = talonavicular joint and calcaneocuboid joint: divides hindfoot and midfoot.
- Lisfranc joint = tarsometatarsal joint: divides midfoot and forefoot.

- Supination = inversion adduction and plantarflexion.
- Pronation = eversion abduction and dorsiflexion.

- Introduce yourself to the patient.
- Ask the patient for permission to perform an examination.
- Adequately expose both ankles and both feet.
- Ask the patient if their ankle or foot is painful.

Patient standing
Look
- Gait (observe patient walking from in front and behind)
    - antalgic: ↓ stance phase;
    - foot drop: high-stepping gait and slapping movement after heel strike;
    - stiff foot;
    - neuropathic, e.g. high-stepping gait in tabes dorsalis due to loss of position sense.

If an abnormal gait pattern is suspected one can also inspect footprint and shoe wear.

Look from in front and behind
- Skin
- Shape
    - swelling (subcutaneous tissue, tendon sheath, joint);
    - wasting (e.g. calf muscles);
    - deformity (e.g. pes cavus/pes planus, calcaneal prominence).
- Position
    - resting position;

- from behind: varus/valgus deformity of heel (normal: slight valgus), alignment of forefoot, longitudual arch.
- Compare with the opposite limb (record pattern of joint involvement, if polyarticular).

Move
- Patient stands on tiptoe
  - normal: heel moves into varus;
  - flat foot: if mobile – medial arch reconstitutes.

Patient supine
Look
- Skin
  - scars;
  - callosities on sole/toes;
  - colour changes (including bruising, pallor, erythema).
- Shape
  - swelling (subcutaneous tissue, tendon sheath, joint);
  - wasting.
- Alignment
  - ankle (e.g. calcaneus, equinus);
  - subtalar joint (e.g. varus, valgus);
  - medial arch (e.g. planus, cavus);
  - forefoot (e.g. metatarsus adductus, metatarsus abductus);
  - toes (e.g. hallux valgus, claw toes).

Feel
Note any tenderness.
- Skin
  - temperature;
  - moisture;
  - sensation (light touch, pinprick, two-point discrimination).
- Soft tissues (lumps, thickening, wasting)
  - Achilles' tendon;
  - peroneal tendons;
  - tibialis posterior tendon;
  - medial and lateral ligament complexes;
  - heel pad;
  - plantar fascia.

- Bones and joints (outlines, synovium, fluid swelling)
  - medial and lateral malleoli;
  - ankle joint;
  - tibiofibular syndesmosis;
  - os calcis (including calcaneal attachment of Achilles tendon);
  - midfoot;
  - forefoot (including sesamoid bones);
  - toes.
- Pulses
  - dorsalis pedis (dorsum of midfoot lateral to extensor hallucis longus tendon);
  - posterior tibial (between medial malleolus and Achilles tendon);
  - capillary refill.

Move

Normal range of movement (*see Diagram 19*)

Passive
- Ankle joint: dorsiflexion (15°) and plantarflexion (45°)
  - hold tibia with left hand, cup heel and hold midfoot in right hand, *or* hold heel in left hand and hold midfoot in right hand;
  - if dorsiflexion restricted, flex knee and repeat;
  - if dorsiflexion restored ⇒ tight Achilles tendon.
- Subtalar joint: inversion (30°) and eversion (20°): hold tibia with left hand and hold heel with right hand then move heel.
- Mid-tarsal joint: forefoot rotation: hold heel still with left hand and move forefoot in rotatory movement.
- Metatarsophalangeal joints: dorsiflexion (50°) and plantarflexion (30°).

Active
- ankle joint: dorsiflexion and plantarflexion.
- subtalar joint: inversion and eversion.

Special tests

- Anterior stress test (anterior drawer)
  - allow foot to fall into slight equinus, stabilize distal tibia with one hand, cup heel in other hand and apply anterior force;
  - *or* rest heel on firm surface and push backwards on distal tibia.
- Inversion stress test (talar tilt)
  - stabilize medial aspect of distal tibia with one hand and apply inversion

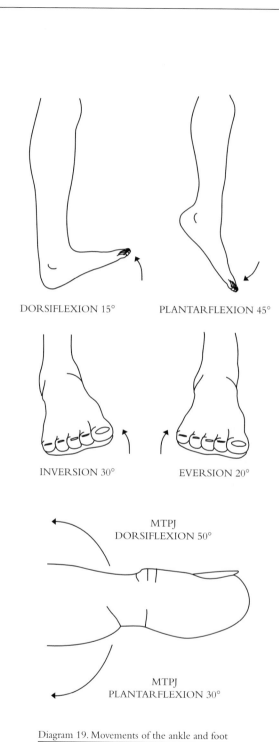

DORSIFLEXION 15°   PLANTARFLEXION 45°

INVERSION 30°   EVERSION 20°

MTPJ
DORSIFLEXION 50°

MTPJ
PLANTARFLEXION 30°

Diagram 19. Movements of the ankle and foot

force to hindfoot with other hand;

- in plantar flexion, tests anterior talofibular ligament;
- in neutral or slight dorsiflexion, tests calcaneofibular ligament.
- Eversion stress test (talar tilt)
  - tests superficial deltoid ligament complex;
  - allow foot to fall into slight equinus, stabilize lateral aspect of distal tibia with one hand and apply eversion force to hindfoot with other hand.
- Peroneal subluxation: attempt to sublux peroneal tendons forwards from behind lateral malleolus.
- External rotation stress test
  - tests syndesmosis and deep deltoid ligament;
  - hold tibia in one hand with ankle neutral;
  - pain on external rotation of foot ⇒ syndesmotic injury (sprain of inferior tibiofibular syndesmosis).
- Squeeze test
  - squeeze leg (fibula towards tibia) at mid-calf level;
  - ankle pain ⇒ syndesmotic injury.

Patient prone
Look
- Shape
  - swelling (subcutaneous tissue, tendon sheath, joint);
  - deformity.
- Position: resting position with foot hanging over end of couch ('angle of dangle')
  - normal: slightly plantar flexed;
  - Achilles' tendon rupture: hangs vertically.

Feel
Note any tenderness.
- Skin
- Soft tissues
  - lumps, thickening, calf wasting;
  - palpable gap in Achilles' tendon (usually 3-5 cm proximal to calcaneal insertion).
- Bones and joints: outlines, synovium, fluid swelling.

Special test
- Simmond's test
  - with feet hanging over end of couch, squeeze each calf in turn;
  - +ve: no passive plantarflexion at ankle $\Rightarrow$ ruptured tendo Achilles.

X-ray

Ankle
- AP.
- Lateral.

Additional views
- Mortise view (AP with foot internally rotated 15°).
- Oblique views (45° internal rotation, 45° external rotation).
- Stress views (with or without local anaesthesia, >5 days after injury): anterior draw, talar tilt
  - anterior draw +ve: anterior subluxation >10 mm;
  - talar tilt +ve: tilt >10° more than asymptomatic side.

Criteria for ankle radiograph
In patients presenting with an ankle injury:
- Deformity, crepitus or instability.
- Bruising or severe swelling.
- Moderate/severe pain on weight-bearing.
- Point bony tenderness on palpation.
- Injury of tendon, vessel or nerve.
- Suspected foreign body.
- Age.

Assessment of ankle radiograph
- Adequacy.
- Alignment
  - AP: talus in mortise (talar shift = lateral displacement of talus);
  - lateral: dome of talus congruent with distal tibial articular surface.
- Bones
  - distal tibia (including medial malleolus);
  - distal fibula (including lateral malleolus);
  - margins of ankle joint;
  - talus.

- Cartilage and joints (joint space, loose bodies)
  - ankle joint;
  - distal tibiofibular joint (diastasis = widening of the distal tibiofibular joint).
- Soft tissues.

Heel (hindfoot)

- Lateral
  - Böhler's angle (normal 25-40°, often ↓ in calcaneal fractures) = angle subtended by lines from posterior tuberosity to superior aspect of posterior facet and from posterior facet to superior margin of anterior process;
  - crucial angle of Gissane (normal 135 and 10°, often ↓ in calcaneal fractures) = angle on superior border of calcaneus articulating with lateral process of talus.
- Axial

Foot

- AP standing
  - hallux valgus angle (valgus angle at 1st metatarsophalangeal joint) >15°;
  - metatarsus primus varus: intermetatarsal angle (between 1st and 2nd metatarsals) >9°.
- Oblique.
- Lateral.

Additional views

- Lateral standing.
- Sesamoid: tangential view (hallux MTPJ injury).
- Reverse oblique (navicular injury).
- Splay (Lisfranc's joint injury).

EXAMINATION OF THE CERVICAL SPINE

- Introduce yourself to the patient.
- Ask the patient for permission to perform an examination.
- Adequately expose their neck (and upper limbs and lower limbs).
- Do not expose external genitalia (consider a patient's privacy in the examination setting).
- Ask the patient if their neck is painful.

Look
- Skin: scars, bruising, lacerations.
- Shape: loss of lordosis, swelling, muscle wasting (in pectoral girdle).
- Posture: deformity: forward flexion, lateral flexion, rotation (torticollis).

Feel
Note any tenderness.
- Skin: temperature.
- Soft tissues: muscle spasm, tenderness, crepitus, 'boggy' sensation.
- Bony points
    - spinous processes: tenderness, step deformity (C7 usually the most prominent);
    - transverse processes (behind carotid artery).

Move
Normal range of movement (*see Diagram 20*)

Can express range of movement in absolute angles or in terms of percentages of normal. Angles may be measured using a spatula held between the patient's clenched teeth as a reference.

Active ± passive
- Flexion (chin touches chest, i.e. chin–chest distance = 0 cm) (65°).
- Extension (occipitomental line 45° above horizontal) (65°).
- Lateral flexion (45° to either side).
- Rotation (80° to either side).

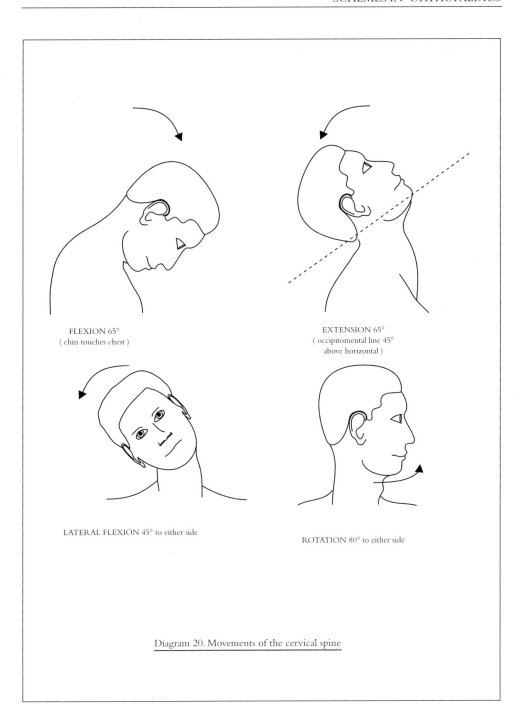

FLEXION 65°
(chin touches chest)

EXTENSION 65°
(occipitomental line 45°
above horizontal)

LATERAL FLEXION 45° to either side

ROTATION 80° to either side

Diagram 20. Movements of the cervical spine

Neurological examination of upper limbs
(See also **EXAMINATION OF THE PERIPHERAL NERVOUS SYSTEM** page 106).
- Power
  - shoulder abduction (deltoid): hold at 90° abduction (C5);
  - elbow flexion (C5/6) and extension (C7/8);
  - wrist flexion (C6/7) and extension (C6/7);
  - finger abduction (T1).
- Reflexes: biceps jerk, brachioradialis jerk, triceps jerk.
- Sensation (test dermatomes in sequence working from distal to proximal).

Neurological examination of lower limbs
(See also **EXAMINATION OF THE PERIPHERAL NERVOUS SYSTEM** page 106).
- Power
  - hip flexion (L2/3);
    knee extension (L3/4) and flexion (L5/S1);
  - ankles dorsiflexion (L4/5) and plantarflexion (S1/2);
  - hallux extension (L5/S1).
- Reflexes: knee jerk, ankle jerk, plantar response; ± abdominal reflex.
- Sensation (test dermatomes in sequence working from distal to proximal).
- Acute cervical spine injury
  - ? priapism ⇒ evidence of autonomic dysfunction;
  - PR: perianal sensation, anal tone, anal reflex, bulbocavernosus reflex.

Special tests
- Cervical disc disease
  - Spurling's manoeuvre
    - head tilted towards affected side;
    - gentle neck extension (or lateral flexion and rotation to affected side);
    - pain (especially arm pain) ⇒ cervical nerve root compression.
  - Shoulder abduction relief test: relief of pain with shoulder abduction ⇒ soft cervical disc protrusion.
- Thoracic outlet syndrome (compression of neurovascular structures in root of neck).

Vascular tests (+ve if obliteration of radial pulse/supraclavicular bruit; high false +ve rate)
  - arm at rest;
  - hyperabduction of shoulder;

- hyperextension of shoulder;
- military brace;
- Adson's test
    - patient sits with hands on knees;
    - neck extended and rotated to affected side or opposite side (modified Adson's test);
    - deep inspiration held.
- Wright's test
    - neck extended and rotated to opposite side;
    - shoulder braced (extended);
    - abduction and external rotation of arm.

Venous congestion of arm if subclavian vein involved.

Neurological tests

- Supraclavicular percussion pain (+ve Tinel sign).
- Supraclavicular thumb pressure (30 s): Spurling's sign = pain produced by direct pressure in supraclavicular fossa $\Rightarrow$ irritability of brachial plexus.
- Weak muscles: triceps (C7), grip (C7/8), interossei (C8/T1).
- Hyperaesthesia to light touch/pinprick (e.g. C8/T1 dermatomes).
- Roos' test (elevated arm exercise test):
    - shoulders braced (extended);
    - arms abducted 90° and elbows flexed 90°;
    - open and close fists for up to 3 min;
    - +ve: reproduction of symptoms (fatigue, cramp, hand/finger blanching, tingling).

Trauma

- The cervical spine should be immobilized in the neutral position (using a semi-rigid cervical collar, sandbags and tape).
- If a cervical spine injury is suspected, examination should be deferred until adequate radiographs have been taken to exclude vertebral fractures.
- Examination should then be performed with in-line manual immobilization of the cervical spine while the cervical collar is removed.
- Movements should only be tested if there are no significant symptoms, the radiographs are normal and inspection and palpation are normal.

Clinical signs of cervical cord injury in an unconscious patient
- Flaccid areflexia, especially with a flaccid anal sphincter.
- Diaphragmatic breathing.

- Ability to flex, but not extend, at the elbow.
- Grimacing in response to a painful stimulus above, but not below, the clavicle.
- ↓ BP and ↓ HR, especially in the absence of hypovolaemia.
- Priapism: an uncommon but characteristic sign.

X-ray
- AP.
- Lateral (may need to apply downward traction on arms to get view of C7/T1 junction).
- Open-mouth (odontoid).

Good quality lateral cervical spine radiograph is mandatory for all major trauma patients.

Additional views
- Swimmer's view (for C7/T1 junction): lateral with arm maximally abducted. Useful if pulling shoulders down does not give view of C7/T1.
- Oblique views (pedicles, articular processes, C7/T1).
- Traction view
    - apply traction via cervical halter;
    - slowly increase weight to maximum of $\frac{1}{3}$ body weight.
- Flexion and extension lateral views
    - to exclude a ligamentous injury in patient with normal standard radiographs but continuing pain/spasm;
    - contraindications: altered state of consciousness, neurological deficit, inability to flex or extend without assistance;
    - flexion and extension movements should made by patient under supervision but with no assistance;
    - head can be supported (e.g. by lead-gloved hand or pillow) after neck flexion has been achieved actively;
    - patient must stop if symptoms worsen.

Alternative imaging
- Tomography.
- CT.

Assessment of a lateral cervical spine radiograph *(see Diagram 21)*.
- Adequacy: seven cervical vertebrae and view of C7/T1 junction.
- Alignment
    - four lordotic curves
        - anterior margin of vertebral bodies [e];

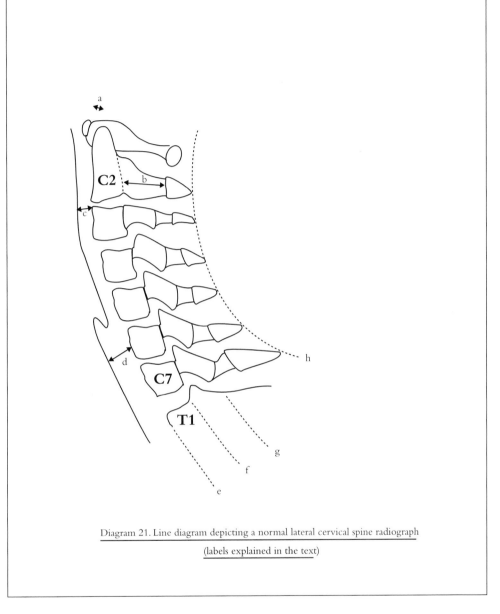

Diagram 21. Line diagram depicting a normal lateral cervical spine radiograph

(labels explained in the text)

- posterior margin of vertebral bodies (anterior spinal canal) [f];
- spinolaminar (posterior spinal canal) [g];
- spinous processes [h].
- widening of interspinous spaces ('fanning') ⇒ torn posterior ligamentous complex.

- Bones
  - vertebral bodies: contour, axial height;
  - pedicles;
  - laminae;
  - spinous processes;
  - odontoid peg;
  - predental space (atlas-odontoid distance) [a]: <3 mm (child 5 mm);
  - width of spinal canal [b]: >13 mm.
- Cartilage and joints
  - intervertebral disc spaces;
  - facet joints;
  - atlantoaxial joint.
- Soft tissues: prevertebral space
  - above larynx [c]: <8 mm ($\frac{1}{3}$ of vertebral body);
  - below larynx [d]: <22 mm (one vertebral body).

Direct radiographic evidence of instability

- ↑ angulation >11° between adjacent vertebral bodies.
- Anterior or posterior translation >3.5 mm.
- Fanning of spinous processes.
- Facet joint widening.
- Rotation of facets.
- Malalignment of spinous processes (AP view).
- Lateral tilting of vertebral body (AP view).
- ↑ interspace separation >1.7 mm on dynamic radiography (traction view).

Indirect radiographic evidence of instability

- ↑ predental space (>3 mm).
- ↑ prevertebral soft tissue space (>$\frac{1}{3}$ of vertebral body above larynx, > width of vertebral body below larynx).
- Minimal compression fracture of anterior vertebral body.
- Avulsion fracture.
- Undisplaced fracture through body or posterior elements.

EXAMINATION OF THE THORACOLUMBAR SPINE

- Introduce yourself to the patient.
- Ask the patient for permission to perform an examination.
- Adequately expose their back (and lower limbs).
- Do not expose external genitalia (consider a patient's privacy in the examination setting).
- Ask the patient if their back is painful.

Patient standing
Look
- Gait.
- Skin
    - scars, sinuses;
    - pigmentation (e.g. *café-au-lait* spots in neurofibromatosis);
    - abnormal hair (e.g. spinal dysraphism);
    - unusual skin creases.
- Shape and posture
    - From behind: scoliosis
        - list to one side;
        - tilt of shoulders;
        - tilt of pelvis (check level of iliac crests);
        - abnormal flank crease;
        - rib hump (most prominent on forward flexion);
        - ? disappears on sitting, forward or lateral flexion, suspension;
        - check leg lengths.
    - From the side
        - kyphosis (gibbus), lordosis, rotation;
        - 'wall' test
            - patient stands flush to wall;
            - spinal deformity often becomes more obvious.

Feel
- Skin: temperature.
- Soft tissue contours: interspinous ligaments.
- Bony landmarks: spinous processes (? step deformity).

- Tenderness
    - between lumbar spines;
    - lumbosacral junction;
    - lumbar muscles;
    - sacroiliac joints.
- Percussion tenderness (in forward flexion).

Move

Normal range of movement *(see Diagram 22)*

Can express range of movement in absolute angles or in terms of percentages of normal.

Active and passive

- Forward flexion
    - composite movement with hip flexion;
    - ensure knees do not flex;
    - check for any scoliosis;
    - measure distance of fingertips from floor (normal <5 cm).
- Extension (30°): ensure knees do not flex.
- Lateral flexion (30°)
    - patient slides hand down outside of leg;
    - note how far middle fingertip reaches down leg (normal 20 cm from anatomical position).
- Rotation (40°: predominantly thoracic)
    - fix pelvis by sitting patient down;
    - patient folds arms across chest;
    - from above observe change in plane of shoulders.
- Chest expansion (at costo-vertebral joints: normal >7 cm).

Special tests

- Modified Schober test (skin distraction)
    - measure of lumbar flexion;
    - two midline marks made on lumbar spine: at level of PSIS and 15 cm higher;
    - should separate by 6-7 cm on maximum forward flexion;
    - skin attraction (measure of lumbar extension): two marks should draw 2 cm nearer on maximum extension.
- Phalen's test (lumbar spinal stenosis)
    - lumbar spine extended maximally for 1 min;
    - +ve: crescendo of leg symptoms (pain, weakness, numbness) followed by relief of symptoms when patient forward flexes, places hands on couch and places foot of affected leg on stool.

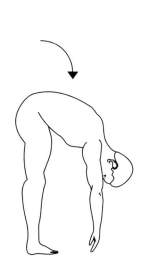

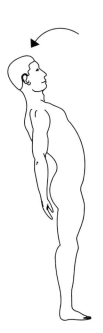

FORWARD FLEXION
fingertips to within 5cm of floor

EXTENSION 30°

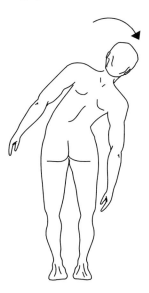

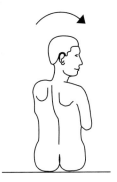

ROTATION 40° to either side

LATERAL FLEXION 30° to either side

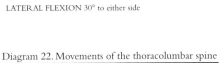

Diagram 22. Movements of the thoracolumbar spine

Patient prone
Feel
- Bony outlines
    - step deformity, gaps;
    - tenderness: facet joints, sacroiliac joints, iliolumbar ligaments.
- Sensation: back of legs and thighs.

Move
- Power: hamstrings (hip extension and knee flexion).

Stretch testing
- Femoral stretch test: lumbar root lesion (L2/3/4)
    - flex knee to 90° and extend hip;
    - +ve: pain in front of thigh and back.

Patient supine
Look
- Shape: muscle wasting of legs.
- Measure: leg lengths.

Move
- Sacroiliac joints
    - 'spring' pelvis (lateral compression);
    - 'open out' pelvis (lateral distraction);
    - Gaenslen test: hyperextend leg (e.g. over side of couch) with pelvis fixed by maximal flexion of opposite hip;
    - FABER test: flexion + abduction + external rotation of fully flexed hip.
- Hip movements (especially if ↑ lumbar lordosis).
- Knee movements.

Stretch testing
- Straight leg raising (SLR): ⇒ lumbosacral root lesion (L4/5/S1)
    - flex hip with knee extended;
    - record angle of straight leg at onset of pain (normal 80°);
    - +ve (Laséque's sign): pain in back of thigh, buttock and back at <60°;
    - hamstring tightness is not significant.

- +ve sciatic stretch
  - extend hip slightly and dorsiflex foot $\rightarrow$ further pain;
  - flex knee $\rightarrow$ relief of pain;
  - pain on plantarflexion of foot suggests functional overlay.
- +ve bowstring test: pressure on lateral popliteal nerve (in popliteal fossa) $\rightarrow$ return of pain.
- crossed sciatic stretch: straight leg raise of unaffected side $\rightarrow$ pain on affected side.

Neurological examination of lower limbs
(See also **EXAMINATION OF THE PERIPHERAL NERVOUS SYSTEM** page 106).
- Tone: including ankle clonus.
- Power
  - hip flexion (L2/3);
  - knee extension (L3/4) and flexion (L5/S1);
  - ankle dorsiflexion (L4/5) and plantarflexion (S1/2);
  - hallux extension (L5/S1).
- Reflexes: knee jerk, ankle jerk, plantar response; ± abdominal reflex.
- Sensation (test dermatomes in sequence working from distal to proximal).

General examination
- Peripheral pulses: femoral, posterior tibial, dorsalis pedis.
- Abdominal examination (including groins): intra-abdominal pathology may present as backache.
- PR
  - perianal sensation, anal tone;
  - anal reflex, bulbocavernosus reflex.

Signs of functional overlay
Waddell criteria for non-organic low back pain:
- ↓ straight leg raise but able to sit up on couch without flexing knees.
- Downward pressure on head (axial loading) or spinal rotation $\Rightarrow$ ↑ back pain.
- Superficial stimulation of lumbar skin (e.g. pinching) $\Rightarrow$ ↑ back pain.
- Non-anatomical tenderness with light touch.
- Widespread (regional) weakness/stocking anaesthesia.
- Over-reaction.

Trauma
- On arrival, ensure adequate immobilization of the entire patient (using spine boards and semirigid cervical collar).
- Following the 1° survey, resuscitation and 2° survey, if there is no evidence of spinal cord injury, log-roll the patient to assess the entire spine.

X-ray
- AP.
- Lateral.

Additional views
- Lateral view of lumbosacral junction: assessment of L5/S1 spondylolisthesis.
- Oblique views of lumbar spine
    - assessment of intervertebral foramina, pedicles and facet joints;
    - useful in spondylolisthesis, unifacet dislocation;
    - identify the 'Scotty dog' shadows
        - nose: transverse process;
        - eye: pedicle (end-on);
        - ear: superior articular process;
        - front leg: inferior articular process;
        - neck: pars interarticularis.
    - 'decapitation' ⇒ spondylolisthesis;
    - elongated neck/'collar' ⇒ spondylolysis.

Alternative imaging
- CT/MRI
    - position of any bony fragments;
    - cord compression/nerve root compression.
- Myelogram.

Assessment of a lateral lumbar spine radiograph
- Adequacy: five lumbar vertebrae and view of thoracolumbar and lumbosacral junctions.
- Alignment: four lordotic curves:
    - anterior longitudinal line;
    - posterior longitudinal line;
    - facet joints;
    - spinous processes.

- Bones
    - vertebral bodies: axial height, contour, density;
    - pedicles;
    - laminae;
    - spinous processes.
- Cartilage and joints
    - intervertebral disc spaces (L5/S1 disc usually narrower than L4/5);
    - facet joints.
- Soft tissues.

Denis' three-column classification of spinal injuries
- Anterior column: in front of middle column.
- Middle column: posterior $\frac{1}{3}$ of vertebral body and posterior longitudinal ligament.
- Posterior column: behind middle column.

Injuries involving more than one column are usually unstable.

Assessment of an AP lumbar spine radiograph
- Adequacy: five lumbar vertebrae and view of thoracolumbar and lumbosacral junctions.
- Alignment
    - vertical alignment of spinous processes;
    - interpedicular distance: progressive $\uparrow$ down vertebral column; interpedicular widening $\Rightarrow$ burst fracture.
- Bones
    - vertebral bodies: axial height, contour, density;
    - pedicles;
    - laminae;
    - transverse processes.
- Cartilage and joints
    - intervertebral disc spaces;
    - facet joints.
- Soft tissues.

EXAMINATION OF THE PERIPHERAL NERVOUS SYSTEM

- Tone.
- Power.
- Reflexes.
- Sensation.

Tone
- Passively flex the limbs through a full range of movement
  - flaccidity $\Rightarrow$ lower motor neurone lesion;
  - rigidity $\Rightarrow$ upper motor neurone lesion.
- Test for wrist and ankle clonus ($\Rightarrow$ upper motor neurone lesion).

Power (see also **Myotomes** below)
- Test each muscle group against resistance
  - look for contraction of muscle or movement of its tendon;
  - palpate muscle belly for contraction.
- Record MRC grade
  - Medical Research Council grading system of muscle power:
    - 0 – no contraction;
    - 1 – flicker of contraction;
    - 2 – active movement with gravity eliminated;
    - 3 – active movement against gravity;
    - 4 – active movement against gravity and resistance;
    - 5 – normal power.
    - Grades 4-, 4 and 4+ indicate movement against slight, moderate and strong resistance respectively.

Reflexes
- Deep tendon reflexes (tested using a tendon hammer)
  - biceps jerk C5/6;
  - brachioradialis jerk C6;
  - triceps jerk C7;
  - knee jerk L3/4;
  - ankle jerk S1.
- Superficial skin reflexes
  - abdominal reflex

- light stroking of each quadrant of abdomen → underlying muscle contraction;
- absence ⇒ upper motor neurone lesion.
- Plantar reflex
    - firm stroking of lateral surface of sole of foot → great toe plantarflexion;
    - extension of great toe ⇒ upper motor neurone lesion.
- Anal reflex (S2-4): light touch (or pinprick) of perianal skin → contraction of external anal sphincter.
- Bulbocavernosus reflex (S3-4): squeeze of glans penis or clitoris, or application of gentle traction to urethral catheter; → contraction of external anal sphincter.

Loss of anal and bulbocavernosus reflexes ⇒ spinal shock or damage to sacral segments of cord. (Do not expose external genitalia in the examination setting.)

Sensation (see also **Dermatomes** below).
- Ask patient to outline area of any sensory abnormality.
- Test each dermatome - work from insensate area to sensate area, or from distal to proximal.
- Two modalities are commonly tested
    - light touch (e.g. cotton wool);
    - superficial pain (e.g. pinprick with disposable pin).
- Can also test two-point discrimination, joint position sense and deep pressure sense.

Myotomes
Myotome = muscle supplied by a single spinal nerve.

C4	diaphragm (respiration).
C5	deltoid (shoulder abduction).
C6	biceps (elbow flexion); biceps jerk.
C7	triceps (elbow extension); triceps jerk.
C8	flexor digitorum profundus (finger flexion); extensor digitorum (finger extension).
T1	abductor pollicis brevis (thumb abduction).
T7-T12	anterior abdominal wall muscles; abdominal reflex.
L1	internal oblique and transversus guarding the inguinal canal.
L2	psoas major (hip flexion).

L3   quadriceps femoris (knee extension);
knee jerk.

L4   tibialis anterior and posterior (foot inversion).

L5   extensor hallucis longus (great toe extension);
peroneal muscles (foot eversion).

S1   gastrocnemius (foot plantarflexion);
ankle jerk.

S2   small muscles of the foot.

S3   perineal muscles
bladder (parasympathetic);
anal and bulbocavernosus reflexes.

Neurological examination conventionally tests muscle groups in sequence

Upper limb

• shoulder abduction	C5
• shoulder adduction	C6/7(8)
• elbow flexion	C5/6
• elbow extension	C7/8
• wrist extension	C6/7
• wrist flexion	C6/7
• supination	C6
• pronation	C7/8
• finger flexion	C7/8
• finger extension	C7/8
• finger abduction	T1.

Lower limb

• hip flexion	L2/3
• hip extension	L4/5
• knee extension	L3/4
• knee flexion	L5/S1
• ankle dorsiflexion	L4/5
• ankle plantarflexion	S1/2
• foot inversion	L4
• foot eversion	L5/S1
• hallux extension	L5/S1
• hallux flexion	S1/2.

Dermatomes

Dermatome = area of skin supplied by a single spinal nerve *(see Diagrams 23–26).*

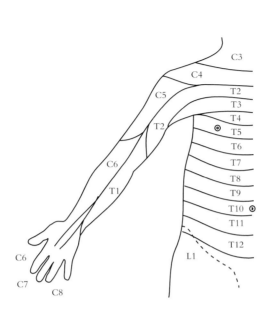

Diagram 23. Upper limb dermatomes (anterior aspect)

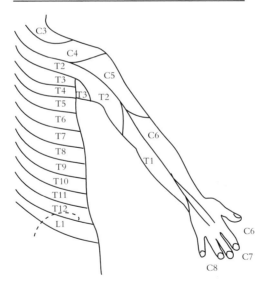

Diagram 24. Upper limb dermatomes (posterior aspect)

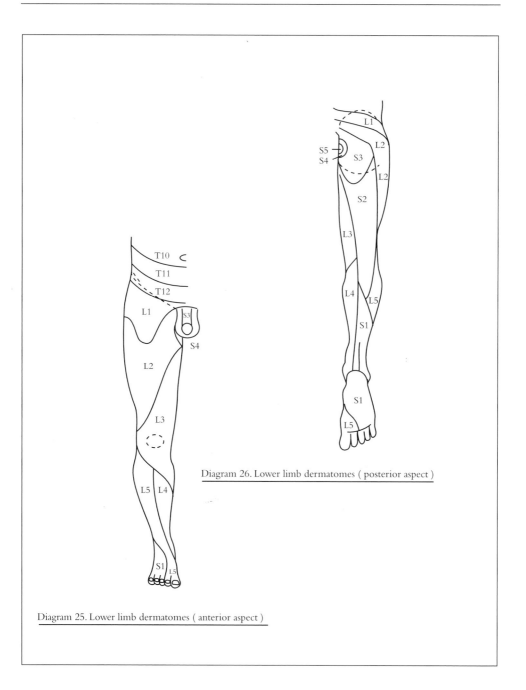

Diagram 26. Lower limb dermatomes (posterior aspect)

Diagram 25. Lower limb dermatomes (anterior aspect)

EXAMINATION OF THE BRACHIAL PLEXUS

Brachial plexus lesions
The classical clinical pictures of upper and lower brachial plexus lesions are:
- Erb-Duchenne palsy (C5,6)
    - ↓ shoulder abduction and external rotation;
    - → adducted and internal rotated arm ('waiter's tip' position).
- Klumpke's palsy (C8,T1)
    - ↓ intrinsic muscles → 'claw hand';
    - ↓ sensation in ulnar part of hand and forearm.

However, brachial plexus injuries are often mixed. Then the site of injury may only be determined by systematic testing of:
- motor function of appropriate muscle groups: active movement against resistance and simultaneous palpation of muscle belly for contraction;
- cutaneous sensation in suitable areas.

Such examination should be structured according to the anatomy of the brachial plexus *(see Diagram 27)*.

Note: individual variation in anatomy is a major pitfall in clinical diagnosis (e.g. digital extensors usually innervated by C8 but they may be innervated by T1, or alternatively all extensors may be paralysed with C8/T1 intact)

Roots
- Dorsal scapular nerve (C5) → rhomboids
    - motor: with arm internally rotated behind back, press palm backwards against resistance.
- Long thoracic nerve (C5, C6, C7) → serratus anterior
    - motor: push against resistance (e.g. a wall) and palpate muscle belly;
    - long thoracic nerve palsy → winging of scapula.

Trunks
- Suprascapular nerve (C5, C6) → supraspinatus and infraspinatus
    - motor: abduction against resistance with arm in 20° abduction and 20° flexion (supraspinatus);
    - external rotation of arm against resistance (infraspinatus).

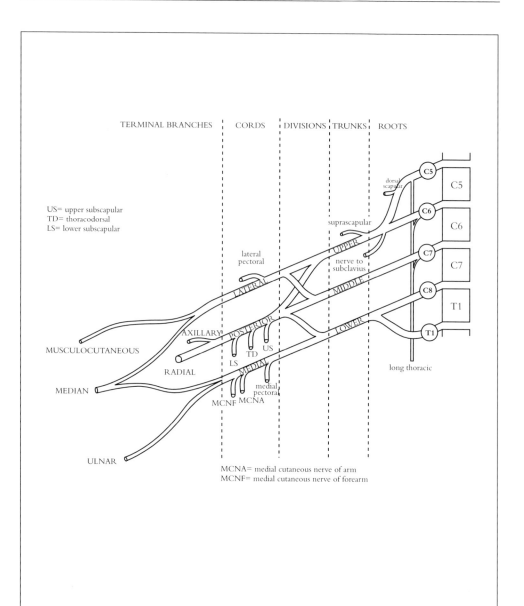

Diagram 27. The brachial plexus

Lateral cord
- Lateral pectoral nerve (C5, C6, C7) → pectoralis major (clavicular head mainly)
  - motor: with arm abducted 90°, push arm forwards against resistance.

Medial cord
- Medial pectoral nerve (C8, T1) → pectoralis major (sternocostal head mainly)
  - motor: with arm abducted 60°, adduct arm against resistance.
- Medial cutaneous nerve of arm (C8, T1)
  - sensation: small area on anterior and medial aspect of arm.
- Medial cutaneous nerve of forearm (C8, T1)
  - sensation: lower part of arm and medial (ulnar) aspect of forearm.

Posterior cord
- Upper subscapular nerve (C6, C7) → subscapularis (upper part)
  - motor: internal rotation against resistance (pectoralis major and latissimus dorsi also used).
- Lower subscapular nerve (C6, C7) → subscapularis (lower part) and teres major
  - motor (teres major): adduct 90° abducted arm against resistance (palpate muscle belly).
- Thoracodorsal nerve (C6, C7, C8) → latissimus dorsi
  - motor: adduct 90° abducted arm against resistance (palpate muscle belly); cough (palpate muscle belly).

Terminal branches
- Axillary nerve (C5, C6).
- Musculocutaneous nerve (C5, C6).
- Ulnar nerve (C8, T1).
- Median nerve (C5, C6, C7, C8, T1).
- Radial nerve (C5, C6, C7, C8, T1).

(See **EXAMINATION OF PERIPHERAL NERVE LESIONS** page 115.)

Pre- and post-ganglionic injuries
It is important to distinguish whether supraclavicular injuries are preganglionic (intradural) or post-ganglionic:
- Preganglionic injury of upper three roots
  - loss of sensation above clavicle;
  - paralysis of ipsilateral hemidiaphragm and serratus anterior and trapezius.
- Preganglionic injury of lower two roots:
  - Horner's syndrome (sympathetic disruption) - ipsilateral pupillary constriction + ptosis and enophthalmos + loss of sweating.

- Post-ganglionic injury:
    - +ve Tinel sign - percussion of posterior triangle of neck → paraesthesia radiating to appropriate dermatome (e.g. thumb/index finger = C6).

- Plain XRs of cervical spine
    - tilting of cervical spine away from side of injury ⇒ complete preganglionic injury;
    - # transverse process C7 or # 1st rib ⇒ preganglionic injury of lower two roots.

EXAMINATION OF PERIPHERAL NERVE LESIONS

(*see Diagram 28*)

Axillary nerve
- Tests
    - motor: abduction against resistance;
    - sensation: lateral aspect of upper arm ('regimental badge' area).
- Lesion
    - ↓ shoulder abduction;
    - ↓ sensation over 'regimental badge' area.

Musculocutaneous nerve
- Tests
    - motor: flex supinated forearm against resistance;
    - sensation: lateral (radial) aspect of forearm.
- Lesion
    - ↓ elbow flexion;
    - ↓ sensation over radial aspect of forearm.

Ulnar nerve
- Tests
    - motor: abduction of little finger;
    - sensation: little finger.
- Low lesion
    - wasting of hypothenar eminence;
    - wasting of 1st dorsal interosseous;
    - 'claw hand' (intrinsic muscle wasting);
    - ↓ abduction of fingers;
    - ↓ adduction of thumb. Froment's sign: flexor pollicis longus used instead of paralysed adductor pollicis to grip a sheet of paper (i.e. IPJ of thumb flexes);
    - hyperextended MCPJs and flexed IPJs of ring and little fingers (paralysed lumbricals and interossei);
    - ↓ sensation over ulnar $1\frac{1}{2}$ digits;
    - Tinel sign: paraesthesia on tapping over ulnar nerve at wrist (in Guyon's canal).

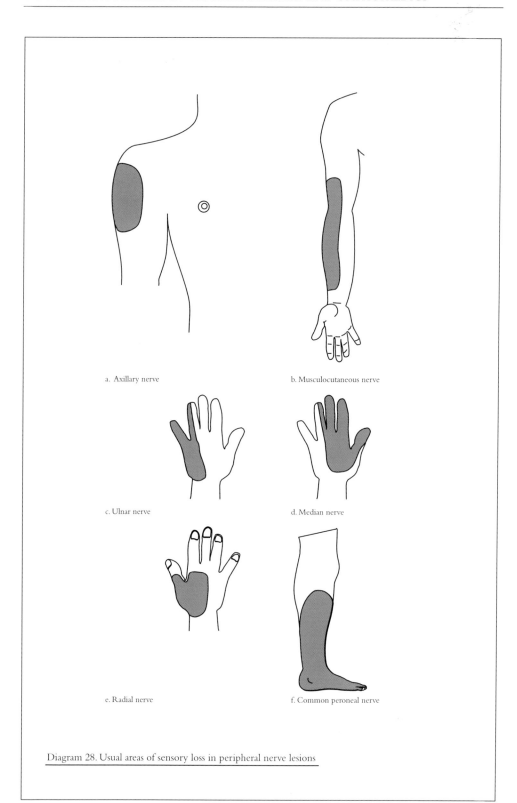

a. Axillary nerve

b. Musculocutaneous nerve

c. Ulnar nerve

d. Median nerve

e. Radial nerve

f. Common peroneal nerve

Diagram 28. Usual areas of sensory loss in peripheral nerve lesions

- High lesion: as for low lesion, plus
  - less marked clawing ('ulnar paradox') due to paralysis of medial $\frac{1}{2}$ of FDP;
  - ↓ sensation over ulnar border of hand;
  - Tinel sign: paraesthesia on tapping over ulnar nerve at elbow (in cubital tunnel).

Median nerve
- Tests
  - motor: abduction of thumb;
  - sensation: index finger.
- Low lesion
  - wasting of thenar eminence;
  - ↓ thumb abduction and opposition;
  - ↓ sensation over radial $2\frac{1}{2}$ digits;
  - Tinel sign: paraesthesia on tapping over median nerve at wrist;
  - Phalen's sign: paraesthesia on keeping wrist in full palmar flexion for >1 min.
- High lesion: as for low lesion, plus:
  - ↓ long flexors to thumb, index and middle fingers (paralysis of anterior interosseous branch of median nerve) → 'pointing index' when trying to clench hand.

Radial nerve
- Tests
  - motor – extension of fingers at MCPJs;
  - sensation – lateral aspect of base of thumb.
- Low lesion
  - ↓ extension at MCPJs (extension possible at IPs using intrinsic muscles);
  - ↓ sensation over lateral aspect of base of thumb.
- High lesion: as for Low lesion, plus:
  - ↓ extension at wrist (wrist drop).
- Very high lesion: as for High lesion, plus:
  - ↓ extension at elbow (triceps paralysis).

Lateral peroneal (popliteal) nerve
- Tests
  - motor
    - dorsiflexion of foot (deep peroneal nerve);

- extension of hallux (deep peroneal nerve);
- eversion of foot (superficial peroneal nerve).
  - sensation
    - lateral aspect of upper half of leg (common peroneal nerve);
    - lateral aspects of ankle and dorsum of foot (superficial peroneal nerve);
    - 1st web space (deep peroneal nerve).
- Common peroneal nerve lesion
  - drop foot;
  - ↓dorsiflexion and eversion;
  - ↓ sensation over anterolateral $\frac{1}{2}$ of leg and dorsum of foot.
- Superficial branch lesion
  - ↓eversion of foot (dorsiflexion intact);
  - ↓sensation over lateral aspect of ankle/dorsum of foot.
- Deep branch lesion
  - ↓ dorsiflexion of foot;
  - ↓ hallux extension;
  - ↓ sensation over 1st web space on dorsum of foot.

EXAMINATION OF A MULTIPLE TRAUMA PATIENT

Adapted from *American College of Surgeons, Advanced Trauma Life Support Student Manual*, 6th edn (1997).

PRIMARY SURVEY AND RESUSCITATION

Airway maintenance and cervical spine protection

- Manual immobilization of cervical spine in neutral (later immobilized by rigid collar and sandbags and tape).
- Assessment of airway
  - verbal response;
    look: agitation, depressed consciousness;
  - listen: abnormal sounds;
  - feel: air movement.
- Establish patent airway
  - clear airway of foreign bodies;
  - chin lift/jaw thrust;
  - oropharyngeal/nasopharyngeal airway;
  - endotracheal intubation (ETT);
  - needle/surgical cricothyroidotomy.

Breathing and ventilation

- Assessment
  - expose chest;
  - check trachea is midline;
  - rate and depth of respirations;
  - unilateral/bilateral chest movement;
  - inspect and palpate for injuries;
  - auscultation (bilateral): anteriorly, axillae, epigastrium (if ETT *in situ*).
- Management
  - 100% O_2 (F_1O_2 >0.85);
  - decompress any tension pneumothorax;
  - seal any open pneumothorax;
  - attach CO_2 monitor to ETT;
  - attach pulse oximeter.

Circulation and haemorrhage control

- Assessment of blood volume/cardiac output
  - level of consciousness;
  - pulse (femoral or carotid artery: quality, rate, regularity);
  - skin colour;
  - capillary refill.
- Identify sites of exsanguinating haemorrhage
- Management
  - direct pressure to any external bleeding site;
  - two large IV cannulae (>16G);
  - 20 ml blood for FBC, U&Es, blood glucose, cross-match, (toxicology), (clotting screen), (amylase);
  - arterial blood gases;
  - warm Hartmann's solution/colloid and whole blood (cross-matched/type-specific/type O);
  - (pneumatic anti-shock garment);
  - ECG (cardiac monitor);
  - urinary catheter and nasogastric tube.

Disability: neurological status

- Assessment
  - level of consciousness (AVPU)
    - A: alert;
    - V: responds to vocal stimuli;
    - P: responds to painful stimuli;
    - U: unresponsive.
  - pupils (size, equality, reaction to light);
  - rapid neurological assessment (tongue out, squeeze fingers, wiggle toes).

Exposure/environmental control

- Completely undress patient.
- Prevent hypothermia (warm environment, warm blankets, warmed IV fluids).
- Log-rolling performed during secondary survey to allow examination of back, rectal examination and examination of posterior aspects of head, neck and limbs.

Further assessment
- Monitoring of vital signs
    - pulse oximeter: heart rate and O_2 saturation;
    - blood pressure (BP);
    - ECG (cardiac monitor);
    - respiratory rate and arterial blood gases;
    - expired CO_2 (monitor attached to ETT);
    - urinary output;
    - temperature;
    - central venous pressure (CVP);
    - blood glucose (finger-prick capillary blood testing).
- X-rays (trauma series): may be performed during secondary survey
    - lateral XR cervical spine;
    - CXR;
    - AP XR pelvis.
- Other investigations to consider
    - diagnostic peritoneal lavage (DPL);
    - abdominal ultrasound scan.

Reassess primary survey and consider need for transfer

SECONDARY SURVEY AND MANAGEMENT
History
- Patient (mnemonic AMPLE)
    - allergies;
    - medications;
    - past medical history/pregnancy;
    - last meal/drink;
    - events/environment related to injury.
- Time of injury
- Mechanism of injury (e.g. from paramedic personnel)
    - blunt trauma: road traffic accidents
        - speed/direction of impact;
        - degree of vehicle deformation;
        - seat belt usage;
        - ejection from vehicle?
    - penetrating trauma (region of body, amount of energy transfer);
    - burns;
    - hypothermia and cold injuries;
    - hazardous environment? (e.g. chemicals, toxins, radiation).

Head–to–toe examination

Head and skull

- Assessment
  - inspection and palpation: scalp and skull, ears, nose, mouth;
  - eyes: visual acuity, pupils (size, equality, reaction to light), conjunctival haemorrhages, penetrating injuries, foreign bodies (remove contact lenses), lens dislocation, fundi (haemorrhages);
  - cranial nerves.
- Management
  - maintain airway;
  - control haemorrhage.

Maxillofacial trauma

- Assessment
  - deformity and tenderness;
  - instability of maxilla ($\Rightarrow$ middle-third fracture);
  - loose/lost teeth.
- Management: maintain airway.

Neck and cervical spine

- Assessment
  - inspection: deformity, bruising, lacerations/penetrating wounds;
  - palpation of cervical spine: step deformity, tenderness, muscle spasm;
  - palpation and auscultation of carotid arteries;
  - lateral XR cervical spine (pull arms down).
- Management: maintain in-line immobilization of cervical spine.

Chest

- Assessment
  - inspection: jugular venous pressure (JVP), bruising, penetrating wounds, deformity, asymmetrical-paradoxical movement;
  - palpation: clavicles, sternum, ribs (anterior and lateral from axillae downwards), AP and lateral compression, asymmetrical movement, surgical emphysema;
  - percussion: anterior, lateral, posterior;
  - auscultation: air entry (high anteriorly, axillae, bases posteriorly), heart sounds;
  - examine posterior chest when patient has been log-rolled.
- Management
  - occlusive dressing (open pneumothorax);
  - pleural decompression: needle thoracocentesis (tension pneumothorax),

chest drain insertion (any significant pneumothorax/haemothorax or following needle thoracocentesis);
- pericardiocentesis (cardiac tamponade);
- endotracheal intubation and intermittent positive-pressure ventilation (pulmonary contusion);
- ECG (cardiac monitor);
- CXR.

Abdomen/pelvis
- Assessment
    - inspection: bruising, abrasions, lacerations, penetrating wounds, movement;
    - palpation: tenderness, AP and lateral compression of pelvis;
    - percussion tenderness;
    - auscultation: bowel sounds, bruits;
    - examine back and buttocks when patient has been log-rolled.
- Management
    - cover exposed bowel with warm saline-soaked pack;
    - exploration of lacerations;
    - (pneumatic anti-shock garment);
    - urinary catheter and nasogastric tube;
    - diagnostic peritoneal lavage (DPL), abdominal ultrasound or CT abdomen;
    - XR pelvis.

Perineal and rectal examination
- Perineal examination
    - blood at external urethral meatus;
    - scrotal haematoma.
- Rectal examination (may be performed after log-rolling patient)
    - perianal sensation;
    - anal sphincter tone;
    - rectal blood;
    - bowel wall integrity;
    - bony spicules (pelvic fractures);
    - prostate position.
- (Vaginal examination.)

Extremities
- Assessment
    - inspection: deformity, bruising, wounds, expanding haematoma;
    - palpation (use rotation and three-point pressure): tenderness, crepitus, abnormal movement;
    - peripheral pulses;
    - distal neurological status: sensation, active movement.
- Management
    - correction of significant deformities (and recheck distal pulses);
    - appropriate splinting of fractures;
    - (pneumatic anti-shock garment);
    - pain relief;
    - tetanus immunization.

Neurological examination
- Assessment
    - level of consciousness: Glasgow Coma Scale;
    - pupils;
    - cranial nerves;
    - peripheral nervous system: sensory deficit, motor deficit, priapism.
- Management:
    - *Spinal cord injury*: adequate immobilization of entire patient (spine boards and semirigid cervical collar).
    - *Head injury*: CT scan (consider intubation + ventilation).

Back
- Assessment (log-roll patient if no evidence of spinal cord injury)
    - inspection: deformity, bruising, penetrating wounds (chest, back, buttocks);
    - palpation ('walk down' vertebral column): bogginess, malalignment, step deformity, bony tenderness, muscle spasm and tenderness.

Investigations
- Diagnostic studies
    - trauma series (lateral XR cervical spine, CXR and XR pelvis);
    - other appropriate X-rays as indicated (e.g. spinal X-rays, extremity X-rays);
    - contrast X-ray studies;
    - CT scans;
    - ultrasound scans;
    - endoscopy.

- Laboratory investigations
    - FBC;
    - U&Es;
    - blood glucose;
    - cross-match;
    - (toxicology);
    - (clotting screen);
    - (amylase);
    - arterial blood gases;
    - pregnancy test: all women of child-bearing age.

RE-EVALUATION
- Response to resuscitation: if not improving, repeat primary then secondary surveys.
- Extent of injuries → priorities for definitive care.
- Check for 'missing' injuries.
- Tetanus immunization.
- Antibiotics (e.g. single dose of a broad-spectrum IV antibiotic for penetrating injuries).
- Pain relief.
- Continuous monitoring of vital signs (aim for urinary output > 50 ml/h or 1 ml/kg/h).
- Frequent re-evaluation during recovery (many more minor injuries are occult initially).

DEFINITIVE CARE
Stabilization and transport
- Rationale for patient transfer: injuries exceed immediate treatment capabilities.
- Transfer procedures.
- Patient's needs during transfer.

RECORDS
- Case notes
    - accurate and complete notes;
    - clear documentation of all injuries;
    - chronological entries.
- Consent for treatment.
- Forensic evidence (save all clothes. significant debris, weapons, etc.).

INDEX

Abdomen 23-27
  auscultation 24
  multiple trauma patient 122-123
  percussion 24
  signs 24-25
  X-ray 25-26
Abdominal mass 25
Adson's test 94
Airway maintenance 119
Allen's test 68
Anal reflex 107
Ankle 85-91
  anatomy 85
  movement 87, 88
  X-ray 90-91
Arteriopath 34-37
  lower limbs 34, 35
Ascites 25
Axillae 17
Axillary nerve 115, 116
Barlow's test 73, 75

Brachial plexus 111-114
  cords 112, 113
  roots 111, 112
  terminal branches 112, 113
  trunks 111, 112
Brachial plexus lesions 111
  post-ganglionic 114
  pre-ganglionic 113
Breast 16-18
  lump differential diagnosis 18
  lymphatic drainage 17
Bulbocavernosus reflex 107

Cardiorespiratory symptoms 1
Cervical disc disease 94
Cervical lymph node drainage 10, 11
Cervical lymphadenopathy 7, 9-10

Cervical spine 92-98
  instability 98
  movement 92, 93
  neurological examination of limbs 94
  protection 119
  trauma 95, 122
  vascular tests 94-95
  X-ray 96-98
Chest 19-22
  auscultation 20
  multiple trauma patient 122-124
  percussion 20
  signs 20, 21
  X-ray 20-22, 26-27
Chronic obstructive pulmonary disease 21
Clubbing 20, 24
Collateral ligaments 79
Common peroneal nerve 116, 118
Congenital dislocation of hip 73
Consolidation 21
Cruciate ligaments 79
  rotatory tests 81-82

Deep tendon reflexes 106
Deformity 44
Dermatomes 108, 109, 110
Developmental dysplasia of hip 73

Elbow 56-59
  movement 57, 58
  secondary ossification centres 59
  X-ray 59
Erb-Duchenne palsy 111

FABER test 102
Finkelstein's test 61
Fistula 32
Foot 85-91
  anatomy 85

movement 86, 88
   X-ray 91
Froment's sign 68

Gaenslen test 102
Gait 70, 77, 85
Gastrointestinal symptoms 1-2
Gauvain's test 75
General surgical symptoms 1-2
Genital tract symptoms 2
Goitre 12-15
Golfer's elbow 57
Grind test 61
Groin 28-31
   swelling differential diagnosis 29

Haemorrhage control 120
Hand 65-69
   anatomy 65
   flexor tendon injuries 68
   grip 65
   movement 66, 67, 68
   rheumatoid 68-69
   X-ray 69
Head 122
Heel (hindfoot) X-ray 91
Hepatomegaly 24
Hernia 28
Hip 70-76
   movement 73, 74
   X-ray 75-76
Hyperthyroidism 14
Hypothyroidism 15

Joint examination 45-47
   movement 46
Joint X-ray 47

Kirk Watson test 61
Klumpke's palsy 111
Knee 77-84
   collateral ligaments 79
   cruciate ligaments 79, 81-82
   meniscal tear 77, 81, 82-83
   movement 79, 80
   X-ray 83-84

Lachman test 80

Larson test 82
Lateral peroneal (popliteal) nerve 117-118
Ligamentous laxity 47
Loss of function 44
Lower limb
   arteries 34, 35
   length discrepancy 71, 72
   multiple trauma patient 124
   neurological examination 94, 103
   pain on walking 37
   ulcer 5-6
   veins 38, 39
Lump 1, 3-4

McMurray test 81
Maxillofacial trauma 122
Median nerve 116, 117
Meniscal tear 77, 81, 82-83
Multiple trauma patient 119-125
   definitive care 125
   head-to-toe examination 122-124
   investigations 124-125
   primary survey 119-121
   re-evaluation 125
   records 125
   resuscitation 119-121
   secondary survey/management 121-125
Musculocutaneous nerve 115, 116
Myotomes 107-108

Neck lump 7-11
   differential diagnosis 9
Neurological examination
   brachial plexus 111-114
   lower limbs 94, 103
   multiple trauma patient 120, 124
   peripheral nerve lesions 115-118
   peripheral nervous system 106-110
   subclavian vein damage 95
   upper limbs 94
Numbness 44

Orthopaedic symptoms 43-44
Ortolani's test 73

Pain 1, 43
Palmar erythema 24
Paraesthesia 44